Who Let in The Sky?

Dear Veeno,

Wonderful to reconnect with you after all these years. Overjoyed to know about your successful kidney transplant. This small and humble book — this labour of love was written when I took TWS in 2010 with Ivan E. Cayote as mentor. At the time I was processing my father's death and the memorialization and cronicling of my memories resulted in this "accidental" book which I had no designs of publishing. But on a whim I submitted the manuscript to Select Books in Singapore and to my delight and surprise, they published this book. Good luck with your creative and personal endeavors.
You are the "Real Deal!"
Love and light always be with you xoxo

Published by Celestial
An imprint of Select Books Pte Ltd
65A, Jalan Tenteram
#02-06, St Michael's Industrial Estate
Singapore 328958
Website: www.selectbooks.com.sg

© Kagan Goh 2012

All rights reserved. No part of this book may be reprinted or reproduced or utilised in any form or by any electronic, mechanical or other means, now known or hereafter invented, including photocopying or recording, or in any information storage or retrieval system, without permission from the publisher.

With the support of

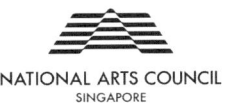

NATIONAL ARTS COUNCIL
SINGAPORE

National Library Board, Singapore Cataloguing-in-Publication Data

Goh, Kagan, 1969-
    Who let in the sky? : a son's tribute to his father Goh Poh Seng's courageous struggle with Parkinson's disease / Kagan Goh. – Singapore : Celestial, 2012.
    p. cm.
    ISBN : 978-981-40-2285-9 (pbk.)

    1. Goh, Poh Seng, 1936-2010 – Health. 2. Goh, Poh Seng, 1936-2010 – Family relationships. 3. Goh, Kagan, 1969- – Family relationships. 4. Parkinson's disease – Patients – Canada – Biography. 5. Poets, Singaporean – 20th century – Biography. 6. Novelists, Singaporean – 20th century – Biography. 7. Fathers and sons. I. Title.

RC382
362.1968330092 -- dc22   OCN759548200

Printed in Singapore

Who Let in The Sky?

A son's tribute to his father
Goh Poh Seng's courageous struggle
with Parkinson's Disease

Kagan Goh

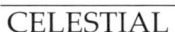
CELESTIAL

Dedicated with Love to My Parents
Goh Poh Seng and Margaret Joyce Wong

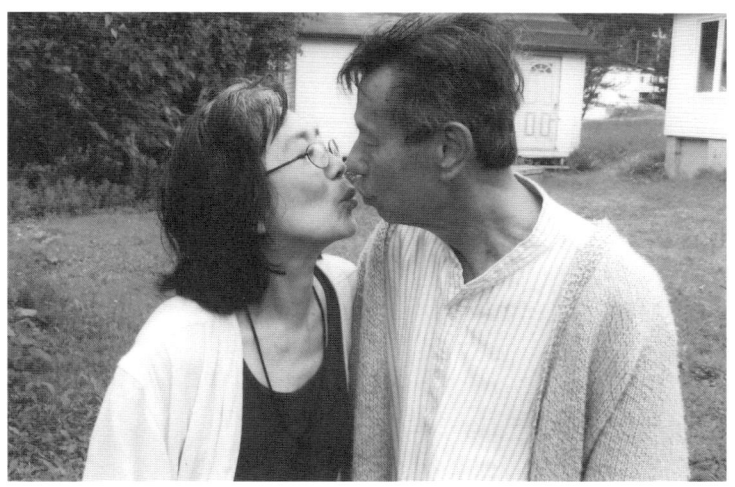

CONTENTS

Goh Poh Seng Biography	09
Foreword By Jamie Reid	11
Parkinson's Disease	20
The Swim	23
Reservations	26
Milestones	31
Comfort Food	34
Inuk Shuk	37
Defying The Hourglass	40
The First Day Back	45
My Sweet Embraceable You	47
The Good Fight	50
Walking Amongst Ghosts	64
God Is Dead	68
Snapshot	71
A Strong Front	72
Beeper	75
Who Let In The Sky?	77
Fields Of Heaven	78
Enter The Dragonfly	81
Acknowledgements	85
About The Author	86

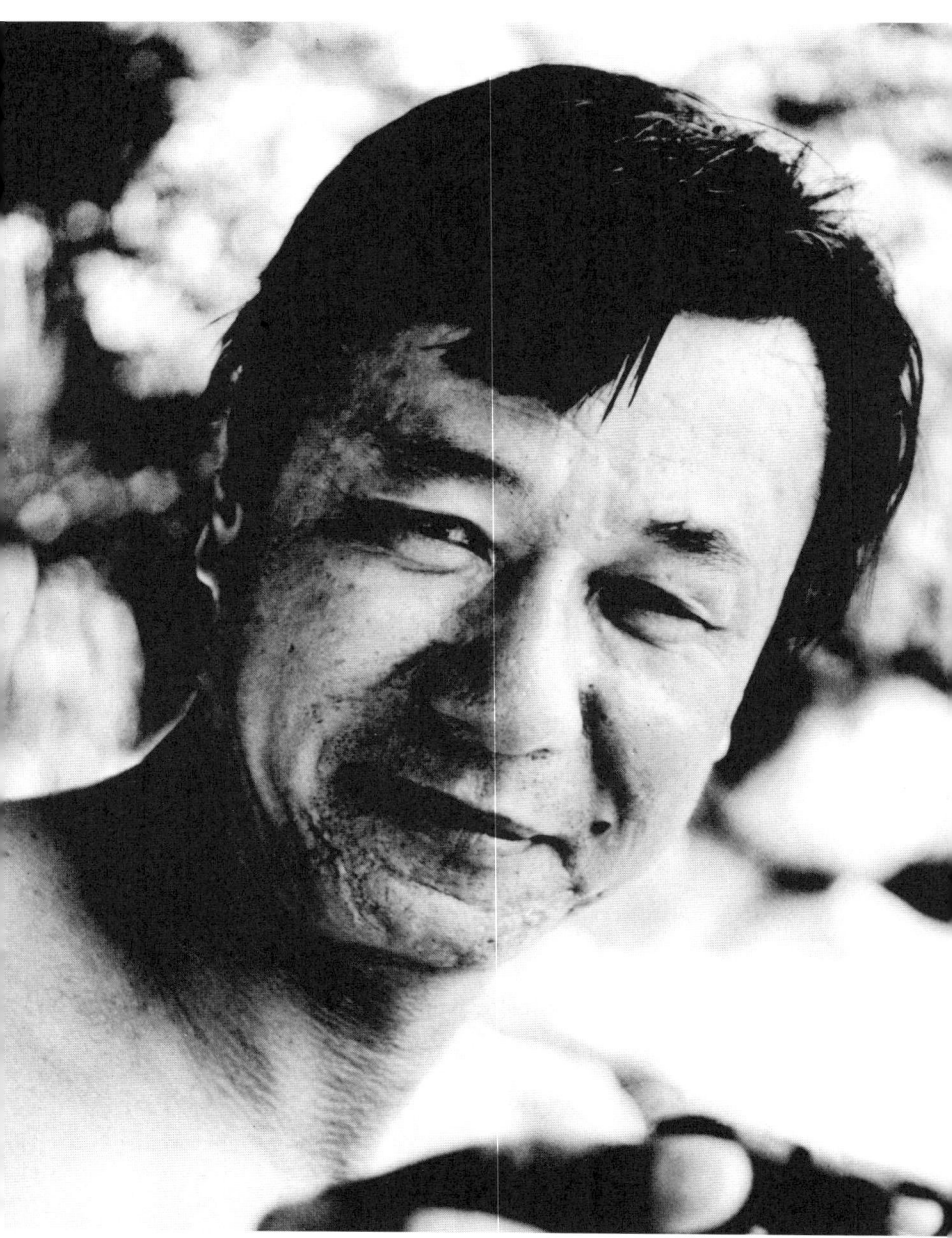

GOH POH SENG BIOGRAPHY

A novelist, poet and playwright, Goh Poh Seng (1936-2010) is regarded as a pioneer of Singapore literature in English. His first book *If We Dream Too Long* (1972) is widely recognised as the first Singapore novel, while his play *When Smiles Are Done* (1965) is one of the first instances of the use of Singlish in drama.

Born in 1936 and educated in Malaya, Goh studied Medicine at University College in Dublin. Goh began writing poetry at 19 while frequenting the pubs of Dublin where he met writers Patrick Kavanagh and Brendan Behan. Encouraged by the publication of his poetry in the university magazine, he wanted to become a writer and at one point dropped out of medical school. He later wrote that "starvation and a love of eating" finally drove him back to medicine.

He settled in Singapore in 1961 to practice as a doctor. In 1967, he was appointed Chairman of the National Theatre Trust and Vice-Chairman of the Arts Council. During his tenure, he laid the groundwork for the formation of the Singapore Symphony, the Singapore Chinese Orchestra, and the Singapore Dance Company. He also organized performances in Singapore for the Bolshoi Ballet, Duke Ellington, Ravi Shankar and David Bowie, giving testimony to his wide and richly contemporary cultural interests and accomplishments.

Goh has published four novels: *If We Dream Too Long*, which won the inaugural National Book Development Council Award in 1976; *The Immolation* (1977); *A Dance of Moths* (1995) which won the National Book Development Council Award for that year; and *Dance*

With White Clouds: A Fable for Grown-ups (2001). While self-actualization and fulfilment are presiding themes in Goh's fiction, his poetry focuses on the lyrical and personal. Goh has authored five volumes of poetry: *Eyewitness* (1976), *Lines from Batu Ferringhi* (1978), *Bird With One Wing* (1982), *The Girl from Ermita & Selected Poems, 1961-1998* (1998) and *As Though The Gods Love Us* (2000). The last two books were published in Canada. Goh received the Cultural Medallion for Literature in Singapore in 1982. His works have been translated into Chinese, Russian, Malay, Tagalog, German, Spanish and French.

In the early eighties, he opened a live music nightclub called Rainbow and a French bistro and jazz venue called Bistro Toulouse-Lautrec where a young Cassandra Wilson got her early start. Original proposals made by Goh also contributed to the eventual plans for the refurbishment of the Singapore River waterfront, which has since become a vibrant, cultural, leisure and tourist centre in the city.

Misunderstood and disillusioned with the authorities, he emigrated with his family to Canada in 1986. There he continued to write and practice medicine, in Newfoundland and Vancouver, until 1995, when Parkinson's disease forced him to retire.

He was writing both poetry and a quartet of stories based on his family, beginning with his grandfather's emigration to Malaya as an indentured labourer, when he passed away in 2010. *Tall Tales and Misadventures of a Young WOG (Western Oriental Gentleman)*, about his student days in Dublin, will be published soon. A collection of the best of his published and unpublished poems is being prepared for publication.

FOREWORD BY JAMIE REID

Kagan Goh's small and modest book provides a brief window into the final years of his father, the distinguished Singaporean novelist, playwright and poet, Goh Poh Seng. In these brief vignettes, Kagan Goh recounts some of the struggles of the Goh family as they deal with the destructive effects of the Parkinson's disease that ultimately ended Goh's productive literary life. As much as anything else, this book is a sincere and touching record of familial devotion and of shared human struggle through grave and finally fatal difficulties. The book provides ample testimony of the strength and love embodied in the Goh family life that has finally seen the family through to a continuing rich life following Goh's death in Vancouver, Canada on January 10th, 2010 at the age of 73.

The brief biography of Goh Poh Seng found on the facing page describes a life filled with activity, involvement and achievement during the 25 years that he lived in Singapore. In this foreword I will concentrate only on his time in Canada when I knew him personally.

In 2007, Goh returned briefly to Singapore after 21 years of self-exile. He went there as the honoured guest of the Singapore Writers Festival. In recognition of his visit, the Singaporean journalist Stephanie Yap wrote a brief précis of his former career in Singapore:

"He was one of the first chairmen of the National Theatre Trust – a predecessor of the National Arts Council – and an entrepreneur who brought British rock star David Bowie to Singapore in 1983.

"A cultural maverick who was constantly earning the ire of the authorities for his boundary-pushing ventures, he also founded the now-defunct Bistro Toulouse-Lautrec, a poetry and jazz cafe, and Rainbow Lounge, Singapore's first disco and live music venue."

Yap continues:

"That year, the authorities shut Rainbow down on the grounds that a member of the house band, Speedway, had made a risque remark in Hokkien while on stage. Suffering heavy financial losses and disillusioned with the conservative climate, he immigrated with his wife and three of his four sons to Canada."

Shocking and devastating as these developments must have been to the Goh family, the end result was that Singapore's loss has been Canada's great gain. With his active and giving nature, Goh went to work in Canada with the same fervor and generosity as he did in Singapore.

Faced with the hard necessity of beginning his life again more or less from scratch, Goh took up the immediate task of upgrading his medical credentials to conform to Canadian regulations in order to be able to make a living for himself and his family in the new country. A medical degree gained from University College in Dublin and his own determination to build a new life were his only passage to the future of his family in Canada.

Once he had successfully completed his qualifying medical exams, Goh embarked on an entirely new adventure. He and his family moved from Vancouver all the way across Canada to Newfoundland, its eastern-most island province. Newfoundland was the only place where he could practice while studying for his final qualifications. Few doctors were willing to work in that remote and isolated place, but Goh came to love Newfoundland as one of his two Canadian homes, separated by the length of the entire continent. Goh became doctor to three small outports or fishing communities in Newfoundland.

With his typical energy he continued to write and rebuild his literary career. His name as a writer was entirely unknown in Canada when he arrived. Armed with an introduction, he contacted Al Pittman, one of Newfoundland's most well-known and loved poets. Al became a close friend and through Al, he met other writers, artists and musicians.

In 1990, Goh received an offer from a private clinic in Vancouver. The family packed and again moved back west.

Goh's first literary appearance of note in Vancouver was in *BC Monthly*, a poetry magazine edited and produced by Gerry Gilbert, a pioneer of the Vancouver literary scene from the 1960s. Gilbert devoted an entire issue to Goh's poem *Tian An Men: Gate of Heavenly Peace*. The poem immortalizes the horrific events in Tian An Men Square in 1989 when the Chinese government ordered the army to shoot down the student protestors. Goh's poem links the events in China with the intense grieving of an outport family for their drowned little girl.

The publication of the poem in Vancouver gave Goh immediate prominence. Many readers of *BC Monthly*, including myself, admired the poem and looked forward to meeting Goh.

My own first encounter with Goh was in 1994 when Gerry Gilbert took me to a party held at his home in Vancouver. There I met his partner Margaret Joyce and all four of his sons, and a host of other interesting people. Thereafter, I attended many pot-luck dinner parties, garden parties and family birthday celebrations year after year at the Goh home in East Vancouver.

The guests at these events were a richly multicultural group of many nationalities. They came from widely separate social circles and age groups: artists, actors, professionals and other culturati as well as some of Goh's close neighbours, crowded together on the balcony of the house and throughout the shady garden in the backyard.

The dinner parties in his kitchen were intimate and smaller affairs. The Vancouver poets: Gerry Gilbert, Billy Little, George Stanley, and Canada's first poet laureate, George Bowering, were frequent participants. The food was plentiful and savoury; curries cooked by the host himself, and "pot luck" brought by the guests, along with a good supply of wine.

I first met C.R. Avery there, a young poet and singer who is one of the leading lights of the performance poetry scene in Vancouver. There, too, I often encountered one of the prima poets of El Salvador, Alfonso Kijadurias. Famous and celebrated in his own country, but barely known in Canada. Shy and unpretentious, Alfonso sang passionately and exquisitely in Spanish, accompanying himself on the guitar to the great pleasure of the other guests.

Indoors or out, the parties often ended with poetry readings in which neophytes and amateurs were received and applauded with as much enthusiasm as the published and well-known poets. On occasion, someone would modestly ask if they could read a poem or sing a song in the language of their homeland: Farsi, Punjabi, Spanish or whatever. These informal readings contributed a great deal to the intellectual and cultural atmosphere of the entire city.

In the years he lived in Vancouver, Goh had gathered around himself an extensive coterie of convivial friends from many countries, and many different walks of life. At the book launch of his first volume of poetry published in Canada in 1998, around 100 people turned out to hear him read. This in a city where 30 attendees at any poetry launch is considered a full success. Even when the effects of Parkinson's disease reduced his voice to a mere whisper, people still turned up to his readings, and received him enthusiastically.

The opening vignette in *Who Let in the Sky?* refers to a poetry reading on Hornby Island, one of the idyllic Gulf Islands between mainland British Columbia and Vancouver Island. It is the only reference in the book to the public readings which Goh continued to carry on in the midst of his infirmity. Hornby Island is a kind of cultural mecca and home to some of the finest and best known British Columbia artists. Jerry Pethick, a truly outstanding post-modern avant-garde sculptor, was a good friend of Goh's as well as Gordon Payne and Tom Burroughs, two fine abstract visual artists.

Kagan's narrative begins more or less with the onset of Goh's infirmity in 1995. It documents some of the intimate moments in the life of the Goh family from that time until Goh's final moments in January 2010. The unabashed purpose of Kagan's book is to memorialize his father. It is therefore written mainly as a family memoir. As a piece of writing for the public, its most outstanding features are its tenderness and its candour. The writing throughout provides touching details of the love and devotion shared between its two main protagonists: father and son.

Like his father, Kagan has the ability to provide the details that establish the intimacy of family relationships. A tender moment between Kagan and his father becomes pure poetry:

"He purses his lips. We kiss goodnight. Even at forty years old, a grown man kissing his father goodnight, pausing to look back at him sink into sleep before turning out the light."

Another passage, terrifying and poignant in beauty, describes Goh's final days:

"Kajin, Kakim and I take turns keeping vigil over Dad, feeding him his favourite food, reading him his own poems. He claps his hands in delight: "Good poem! Good poem!" His mind is reverting to a child-like state. During the night he calls for his childhood servants and deceased relatives, talking to them as if they are present in the room."

The simplicity of the writing allows harsh and distressing truths combined with humourous sentiment, to soften the tragedy of the moment.

Kagan's narrative documents the catastrophes that fell on Goh and his family one after another: a crippling depression followed by the diagnosis of Parkinson's disease.

In the midst of this illness, Goh successfully underwent surgery for colon cancer and the anxiety of a false brain tumour diagnosis. In the last three years of his life, he suffered a number of bouts of aspiration pneumonia. Any single incidence of the pneumonia could have ended his life, but Goh seemed to spring back from each incident with hearty resilience.

As if all of that were not enough, as Goh grapples with frightening daily falls from low blood pressure, increasing hallucinations, and occasional bouts of dementia interspersed with sudden clarity. During his final days, his wife was also suddenly rushed to hospital with a life-threatening ruptured aortic aneurysm. Miraculously, she survived. Kagan's memoir includes an account of a wrenching meeting in the hospital between Margaret Joyce and her husband.

Kagan outlines all of these disasters soberly but tenderly, without flinching from revealing some of the less attractive character traits of his father, especially his self-willed stubbornness. The facts and the responses of the family as reported in the text are allowed to speak for themselves, without unnecessary embellishment in the writing. They resonate all the more touchingly on that account.

Goh's faults, if they can be labeled faults, flow out of his greatest virtue, his unquenchable desire to live his life as fully and completely as possible without holding back. Because it is intended as an account of his father's spirit and courage in dealing with Parkinson's, Kagan's account cannot, does not, recount Goh's ongoing courage to belong and participate in the wider world of his friends and literature at large.

The evidence of that towering effort are seen in the fact that even in the midst of the Parkinson's disease diagnosis, the accompanying depression, and each successive life-threatening incident that followed, Goh was still able to publish two new novels and two new collections of poetry within 15 years, while continuing to work on other unfinished projects as well.

His friends in Vancouver wonderingly watched him bounce back from one life-threatening event after another, continuing to make efforts to resume his former life with an unrelenting stubbornness and resolve. I myself remember one occasion after he returned home weakened by a bout of pneumonia. He called me up to come and visit him, sounding weak and vulnerable on the telephone, so much so that I could barely hear his weakened voice.

The following day, when I responded to his call, I arrived at his home only to find him in the yard in the sunshine in his shorts, enthusiastically mowing the lawn with an old-style push-mower.

Every month or so during the last two years of his life, he would call up a group of friends and put together a lunch or a dinner party. There was no use refusing on account of his health because it had already become clear to us, if not to Goh himself, that his time was limited, and that we had to respond to his calls if we hoped to see him again alive - which he always triumphantly was.

His voice would be a mere whisper, and his gait would be uncertain, but he was always fully present, ready to eat the food that we ordered from restaurants, to enjoy the wine, and to carry his own end of the conversation. He often amused us with stories about his student days in Dublin, where he had met many famous literary figures like the poet Patrick Kavanagh and the playwright Brendan Behan.

The last years of his life were also spent in trying to put together his large collection of unfinished and unpublished manuscripts, to put his life's work into some kind of order. It was sometimes pitiful and disheartening to watch him picking through the notes and papers with his shaky, weakened hands. Nothing daunted, he persevered until the work finally became too much for him.

The present volume is part of the effort to preserve the literary legacy of Goh Poh Seng for the benefit of Singaporean and Canadian readers. Through Goh's estate, his family will be continuing to work for the publication and promotion of his work. New editions of some of his earlier novels are already on the shelves or on their way to publication. A book of previously unpublished stories entitled *Tall Tales & Misadventures of a Young WOG (Western Oriental Gentleman)* is already well under way, along with plans for the publication of his plays, and a collected edition of his poems old and new, for an international audience.

Goh's eldest son, Kasan Goh, has also written a book on his relationship with his father, entitled *Star*, which may find publication soon, as well. The richness of the legacy of Goh Poh Seng, Singapore's first novelist in the English language, will continue to grow.

Jamie Reid (Poet and Friend)
2011

PARKINSON'S DISEASE

All that space
    to negotiate
but the medium's
    no longer air.
It has thickened
    into treacle,
and trapped like a fly,
    it's so hard
    to move.
The struggle
    saps my strength.

    All my life
    I'd wanted
    To be a bird!

Goh Poh Seng
Vancouver,
June, 1999

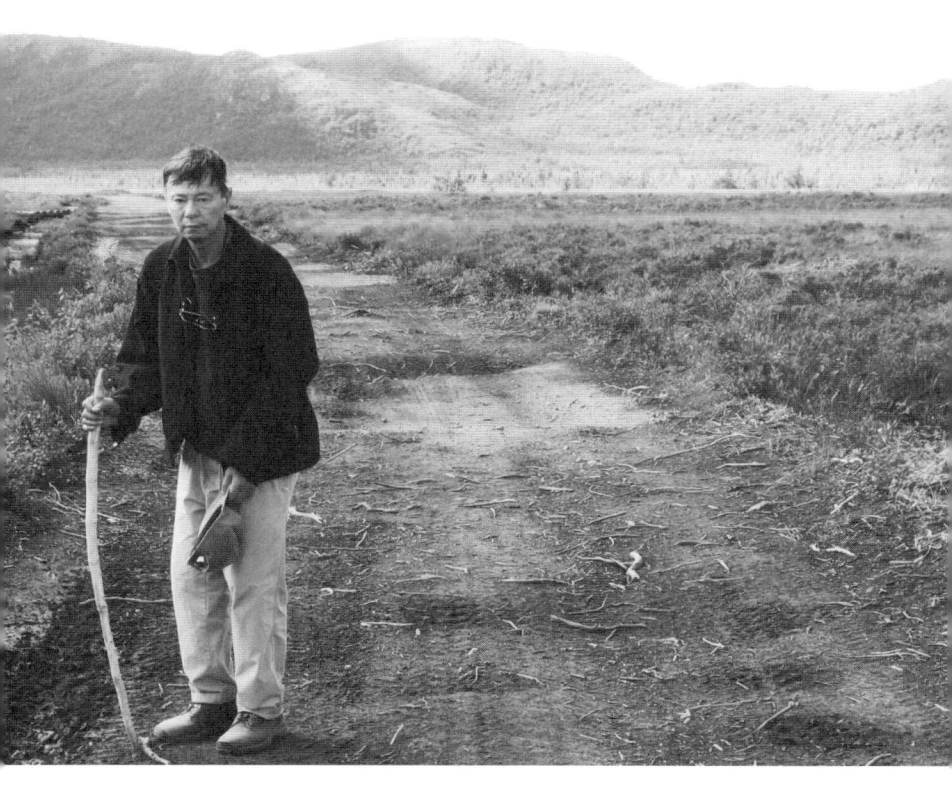

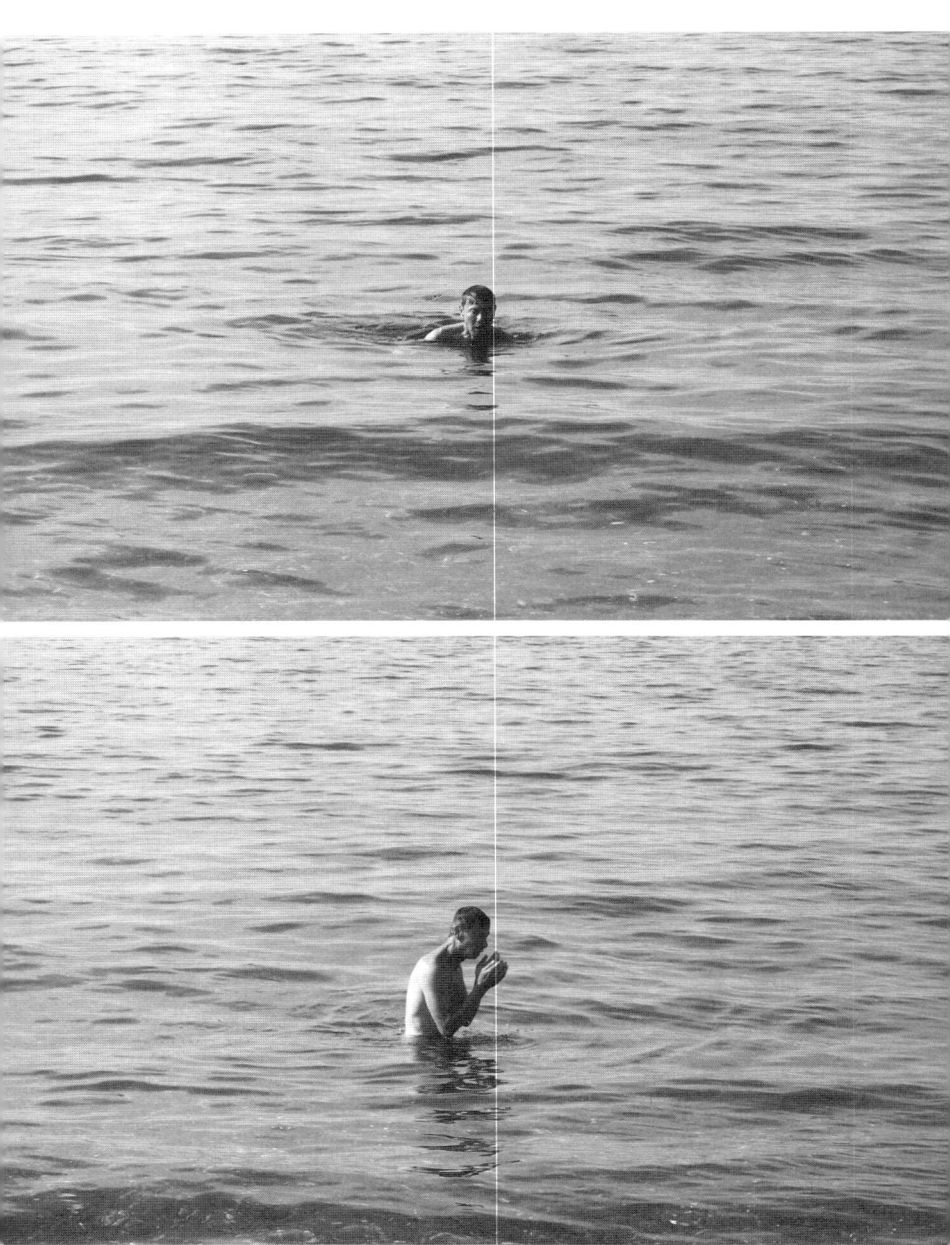

THE SWIM

Dad, Mum and I are on a trip to Hornby Island; one of the northern Gulf Islands parallel with Vancouver Island's Comox Valley. A small community of a thousand residents is distributed across the island, composed of bohemian artists and hippies, many of them American draft dodgers from the Vietnam war, who have chosen to live off the grid.

Dad and I are about to give our first public poetry reading together. My father is the poet Goh Poh Seng, and having inherited his love for poetry, I am following in his footsteps. This reading will be my public debut as a poet in my own right. Having time to spare on the way to the reading, my father pulls our car up to a lake. We decide to take a swim.

I dive into the lake and swim a hundred meters from shore, careful to avoid the dangling reeds below. Do not want to get tangled and drown. The water is warm and pleasant. I see Dad strip and step gingerly into the lake. He paddles towards me doggy style. I swim back towards him for I am quite far out. When he is near he tells me that his medication for his Parkinson's disease is wearing out, his muscles are becoming stiff.

Parkinson's is a degenerative disorder of the central nervous system. It affects my father's movement. He often shakes uncontrollably, suffers from rigidity and walks with a slow gait. Aware of this, I begin to panic as Dad struggles, churning muddy waves that disturb the lake's placid surface.

I say: "Dad, are you OK? Do you need my help?"

He declines: "No." Too proud to accept help from anyone, even from his son.

"Well, let me know if you need me."

We swim back slowly. I swim close to him, alarmed as he struggles; half drowns to get back to shore. I am prepared, poised in case he sinks. He is gulping down mouthfuls of water.

Seeing him struggle reminds me of how I learned to swim as a child. Too short to touch the bottom of the pool, my instructor would hold his hands out to me as I struggled to reach him. He'd walk backwards forcing me by sheer survival instincts to swim the entire length of the pool. Survival is just out of reach yet close enough so I will not drown.

They say parents revert to a child-like state when old. A slow reversal of roles. The reluctant changing of the guard. Awkward and embarrassing. I will never condescend or treat my parents like young children. I only want them to know they can count on me if they need me.

At last we reach the shore and climb out from the muddy bank onto a mossy log. Mum greets us as my father and I towel off.

"How was your swim?" she asks, cheerfully.

"Drank lots of muddy water," he jokes. "Full of vitamins."

We all laugh together. Dad half drowns to get back to shore and jokes about drinking vitamins, as if nothing has happened. I shake my head. That's my Dad.

We pack into the car and drive off to read together for the first time.

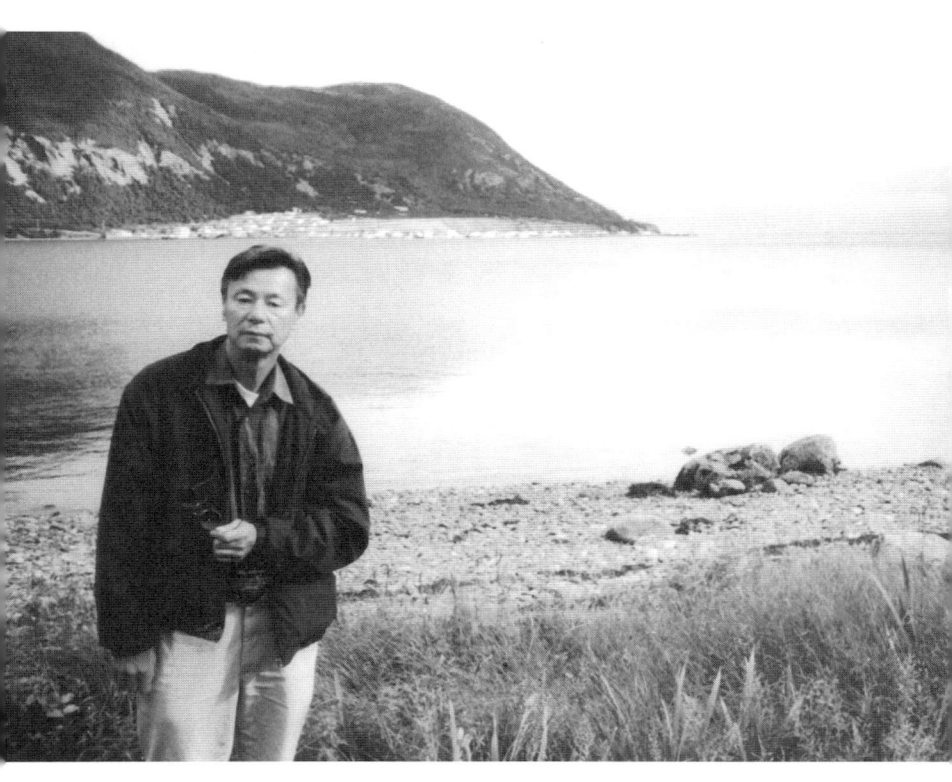

RESERVATIONS

If there is a God,
I wish he is just like my father
for I know no other living soul
so full of gentle loving kindness.
He is my best friend.
He has Parkinson's disease.
He lives in pain,
but he rarely complains.

Gentle as a turtle in his rigid shell
I would sacrifice anything for him to be well.
We make an odd couple.
He nursing my mind.
Me massaging his body.
He, with his Parkinson's.
Me, with my manic depression.
My mind a runaway train
traveling in every direction.

I am thirty years old
but we still kiss each other goodnight.
Lingering, reluctant to part.
As I descend the stairs,
I pray that tomorrow he will still be there.

There is no one I trust more completely.
I have placed my trust in God
but even He has disappointed me.
My father has always been around
when God was nowhere to be found.

Call me a blasphemer.
I can live without God,
but not without my father.
We have so much love to deliver
before the sap in our veins dries up and withers.

If I could I would strike a bargain with Death
to let me take my father across to the other side.
In exchange I would happily give up my life
to be his constant companion.

I have made the reservations.
Booked two first class tickets.
Two reckless sentimental fools,
we have withdrawn all our life savings.
We've emptied our bank accounts
and intend to go on a spending spree,
buying up all the sales on happiness
we can afford from here to Eternity.

Do not worry,
we plan to have a jolly good time.
We have got so much life to burn,
put us in the same urn,
scatter our ashes
and watch us blow
our misfortunes to the wind.

Psychiatrist's report on Kagan Goh, 1999:
"In August he began to feel fearful, sad and tearful. He was afraid of losing his loved ones and would prefer to die vicariously on their behalf. He would not harm himself but the thought of suicide did cross his mind."

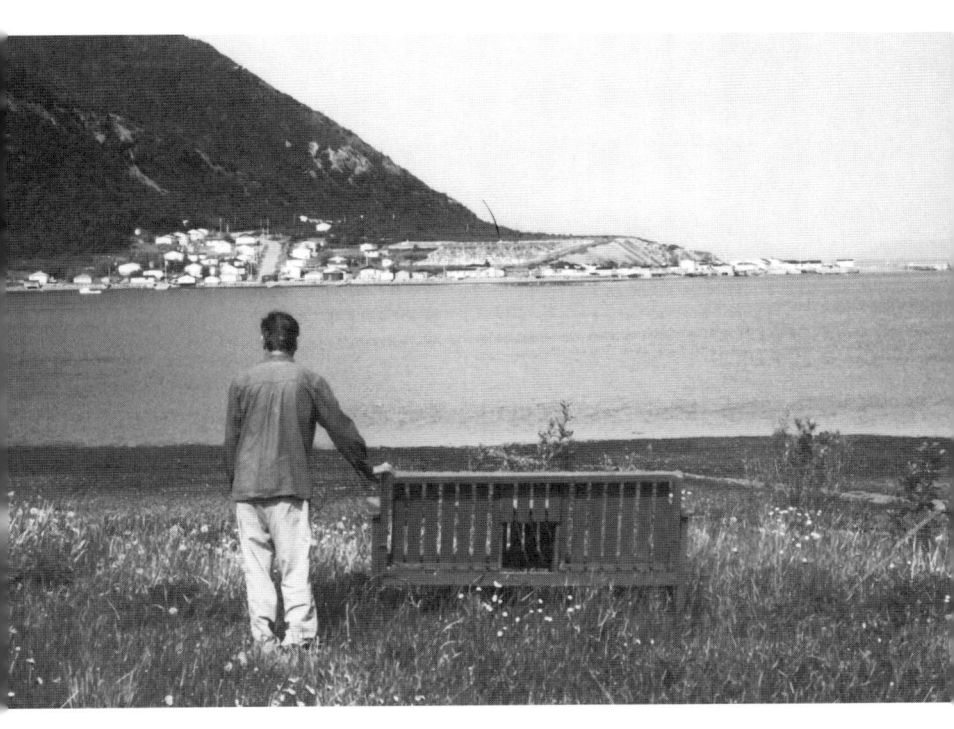

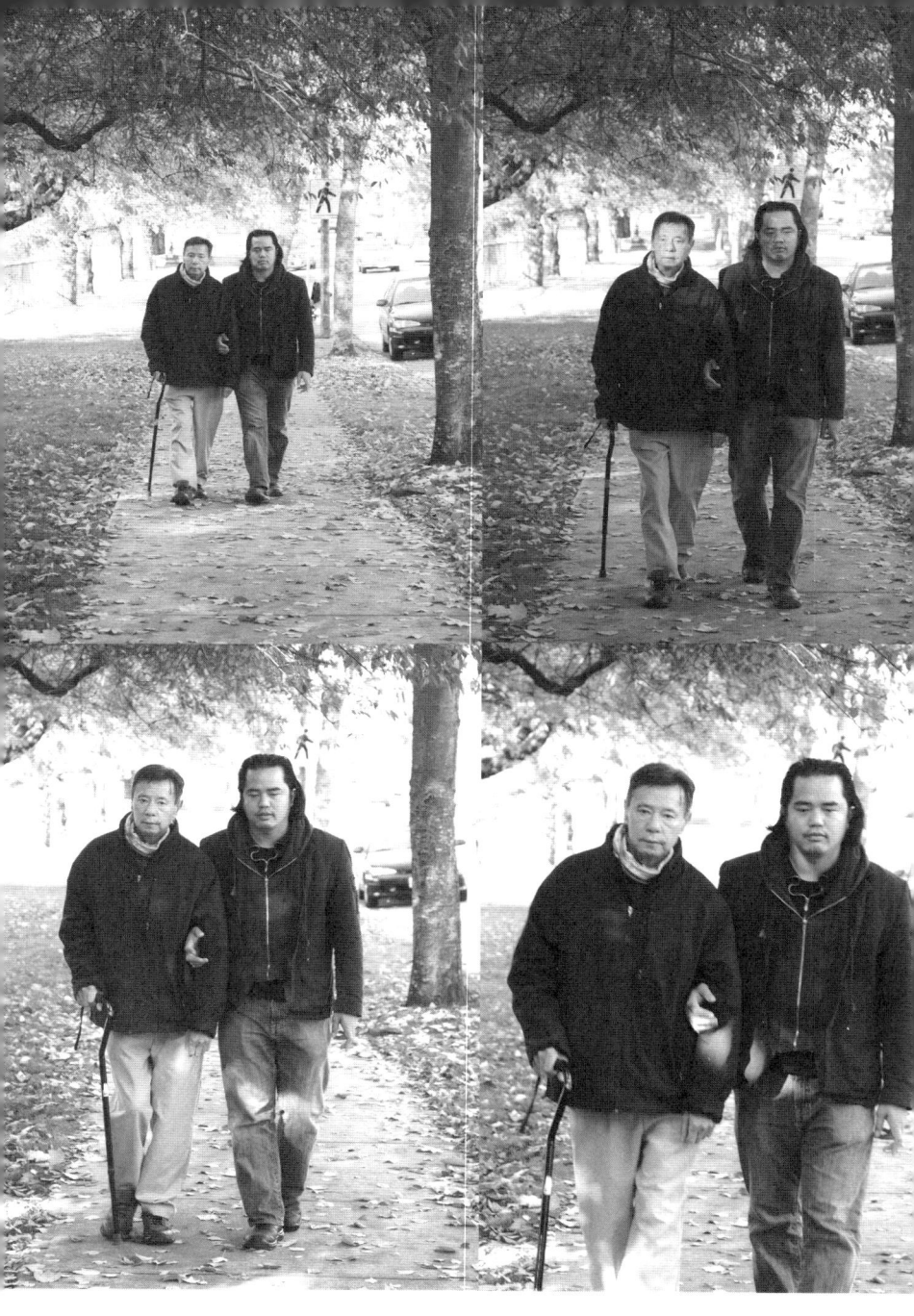

MILESTONES

When I walk with my father
I have to consciously slow down,
temper my impatient fires,
rein in the instincts of my youth
to sprint ahead to the future.

Milestones behind
my father moves in slow motion
mired down by Parkinson's.

He wishes he could dance and soar
free as the bird he cannot be anymore.
My father is jealous of things I can do.
Take for granted.

Some days I roar with rage.
Mind bullying body,
racing beyond the speed limit of sane thought,
running through the red lights of reason.
The broken glass of the past left behind.

My father stumbles to keep up
with my relentless restlessness.
Scared stiff, he shakes from fear

that I may harm myself.
Running so fast I lose insight
unable to tell wrong from right.

I run him ragged,
into the ground,
into the grave.
Why rush, for at the end of the road,
our final milestone, the gravestone awaits?

Perhaps the reason
why my father walks so slow
is he is not yet ready to go.

Not for fear of death.
More so he is too fond of life.

In his eyes
each sunrise and sunset,
each cloud,
each raindrop,
each snowflake,
each fresh morning dew,
each spike of Marram grass
startlingly beautiful.
Miraculous!

I slow down my pace,
taking my sweet time
to walk leisurely with my father.
Slowing down each step as life moves too fast.
Savouring each step as if it is his last.

Vancouver, 1998

COMFORT FOOD

Casually, father tells me he might have a brain tumor. His doctor wants to do M.R.I. (Magnetic Resonance Imaging) in order to confirm or lay to rest our worst fears.

God, please give father a break. He has suffered from depression, Parkinson's and now this. How much suffering can a man take?

He breaks the news so optimistically as if to cheer us up. All my personal problems are but a splinter in God's thumb. I am numb. Nothing matters.

Incomprehensibly he is in good spirits. The fresh air, the long walks in Newfoundland have rejuvenated him. Despite his Parkinson's his mobility is much improved.

There is a long waiting list for M.R.I.s: six to nine months. In six to nine months he could be dead!

At dinner father tries to make light of a morbid subject: "Should I be buried or cremated?"

"Cremation is the way to go," I suggest. "The chemical formaldehyde used to embalm our bodies pollutes the soil with toxins. All for the sake of looking good. Whom are we trying to impress? Grave robbers? We are better use as food for worms."

"Perhaps I could make mince meat of my body," my father adds, getting into the spirit. "It would go nicely in a spaghetti bolognaise sauce. Or I could use my ground up meat in my famous homemade dish: Roti Barbi. Fry finely chopped onions and garlic. Sauté in a frying pan till golden brown. Add my minced meat, mushrooms and a dash of Lee and Perrin sauce. Add curry spices. Fry till done. Layer onto French toast. Wallah! Roti Barbi!"

Mother is disgusted. "Why do we have to bring up the most disgusting topics at the dinner table?"

There is something comforting about discussing the disgusting at dinner. Disgusting conversation with comfort food.

Once when mother was away, father missed her so much that I was sent on an errand; a quest across town to buy plain porridge with codfish from his favorite Chinese restaurant "Daimo." The food brought him comfort. I wonder did he miss Mum or her cooking more?

I confess to mother: "I will miss Dad when he dies. I will miss the both of you. I will be lost without you."

"A person only dies when they have given up on life," she says wisely. "Don't worry, your father has still a lot more living to do. He's not dead yet!"

The M.R.I. waiting list is six months long. We pray for a miracle and God answers our prayers by bumping Dad up the queue to two weeks.

About the test, father said it was like putting his head inside a giant washing machine.

We wait anxiously for the results. Unnecessary phone calls are forbidden as we wait for my father's fate to call. Mother chain smokes. At last, fate calls. We accept the telephone charges. Father does not have cancer.

Thank God! Father suddenly sags. His courage has been bolstering our spirits, as he fought to remain strong for all of us, but in the end he is the frailest of us all.

Taking comfort in the good news, we go out for dinner to celebrate. Mother insists, "No talk about death!"

We go for Chinese food at "Daimo." Mmmm. The food is like home cooking. Famished, father reaches for a second helping.

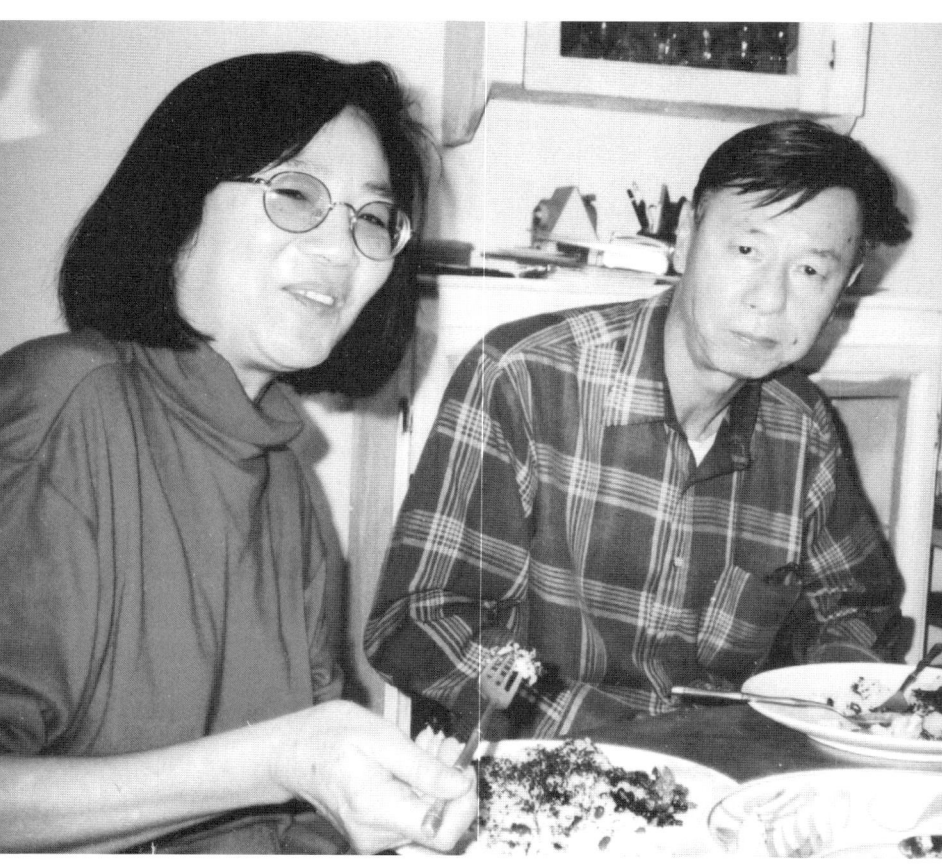

INUK SHUK

My father has been a healer, a physician all his life. Why have none of his sons followed in his footsteps? I can't speak for my brothers, but I am a coward when it comes to pain. As a child, the mere thought of the jab of a needle sent me into hysterics.

My Dad, the hero, saving lives. Once while working hospital shift, a six-year-old child had a hemorrhage and was bleeding to death after a tonsil operation. My father plunged a scalpel into the child's chest, broke open his ribs and massaged the child's heart with his bare bloody hands. His effort failed. The child died. An article was written in a newspaper about my father's "heroic measures" to save the child.

Unfortunately, heroes are not invincible. My father was diagnosed with the double whammy of Parkinson's disease and major depression. His depression was so bad he felt suicidal. I accompanied him as he admitted himself to Saint Paul's Hospital's psychiatric ward, a place I myself would eventually visit more times than I care to remember. My father and I share the bond of being mental health survivors; war veterans keeping each other company as we wander lost through the battlefield of our fractured minds. Walking down the antiseptic fluorescent lit hospital corridors for E.C.T.: Electro Convulsive Therapy, I felt him tremble all over even as he reassured me that electric shock treatment would help his depression.

"It is not as barbaric as the movies make it out to be," he said, unconvincingly.

An optimist even in the worst of circumstances, it seemed to me he was a condemned man who upon sitting on the electric chair, jokes: "Hmmm, it is quite comfortable."

My Dad was strapped down, teeth gritting the bit so he would not bite off his tongue. My father, a human lightning rod, was struck by a thunderbolt from God. A 1000 kilowatts of electricity jolted through his 40-watt body.

After his treatment the doctor complimented him: "You had one hell of an impressive convulsion."

Afterwards, my father and I walked in silence towards the beach at English Bay. We approached the Inuk Shuk monument. Granite slabs of rock arranged to form a mighty statue of a man. It towered over us; arms reaching out to the sea like a vast mother.

Everyone has his own unique threshold of suffering. How much pain can a person endure? As a child, the mere mention of the jab of a needle sent me into hysterics. I am no longer a child and I have endured my fair quota of suffering, but my greatest pain was witnessing helplessly as my father endured the merciless onslaught of Parkinson's. Over time I have witnessed his body harden rigor mortis stiff as granite rock, his muscles rigid, his movements slowed down and laboured. Parkinson's is a cruel disease. The mind remains sharp and lucid while the body decays, falling apart like an ancient ruin. Yet my father embraces life, not unlike the Inuk Shuk that acts as a direction marker, a beacon of hope to those who are lost on the vast, featureless tundra. With arms outstretched he embraces life braving the elements as time slowly erodes his body.

I stood next to my father, looking out into the sea on that cold gray day in English Bay, the wind and rain pelting our faces. What consolation, what words of succor could I say in the face of hopelessness and despair except: "Father, you are not alone."

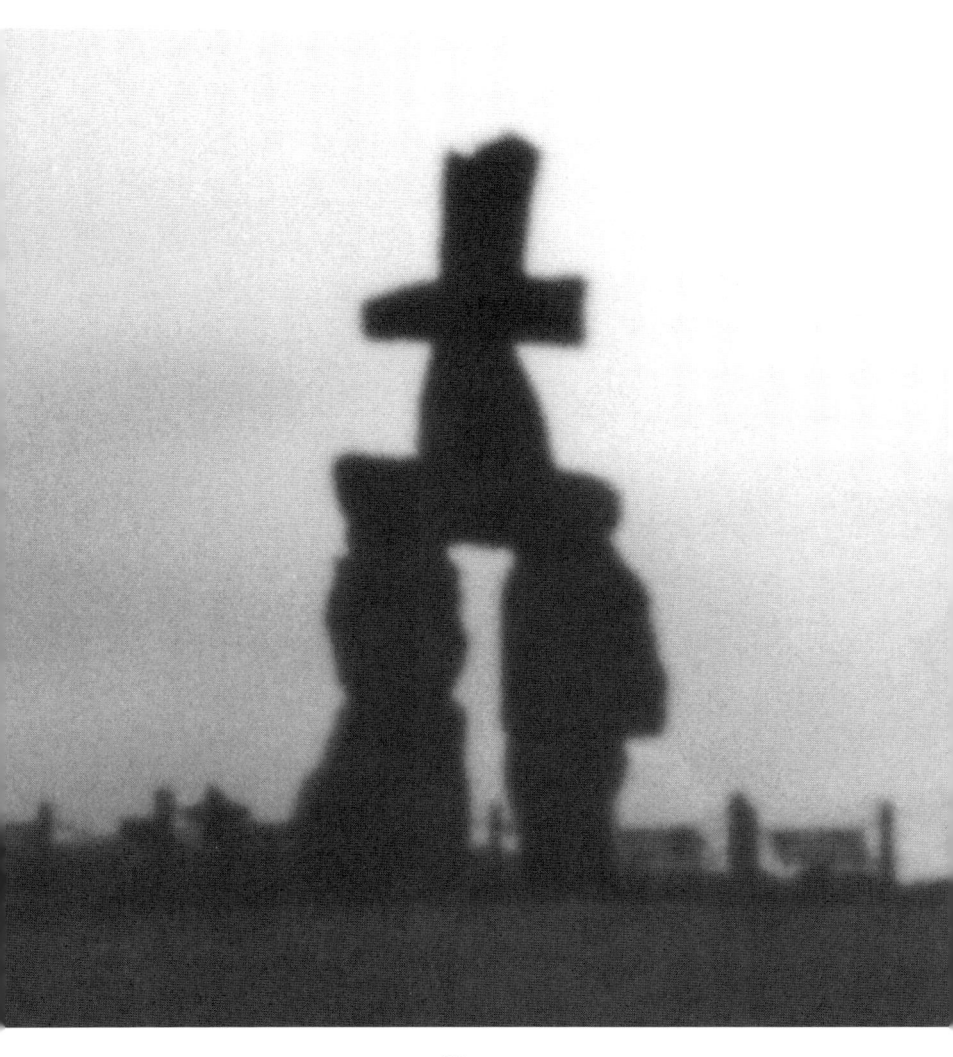

DEFYING THE HOURGLASS

The doctor speaks but I can't hear a word of what he says. There is a ringing in my ears. I feel like my head is submerged underwater. I want to drown out the truth. He points to the X-rays, suddenly, sound rushes in.

"I'm sorry. I wish I had better news to give you."

"How bad is it, doctor?" asks father.

"It doesn't look good. The colonoscopy reveals the cancer has spread throughout the lower colon."

"Oh dear." Mother reaches out and clutches father's hand.

"There is no question, surgery will be necessary. As far as I am concerned, the sooner we operate, the better."

The doctor books an operation for father in two weeks. Leaving the clinic, the three of us are numb with shock. Mother is the first to break the silence. "Oh Sweet, first depression, then Parkinson's, and now this? When is it going to let up? When are we going to get a break?"

At home, I retreat in despair and silence to my room. I bury myself under the blanket to dream the bad news away. Father enters the room.

"Can I come in?"

He sits on the bed. I feel the bed sag from his weight. He pulls the blanket from over my head, places his hand on my shoulder and gently rouses me from my numbed state.

"How are you doing?"

"Fine," I lie, rubbing my eyes. How can anything ever be fine after this?

"I have something important to talk about with you," he says with dead seriousness. He has the demeanour of a man facing his mortality.

"What is it Dad?"

"I may not have much time left."

"Don't say that."

"Listen to me, I need your help. Will you help me finish my memoirs?" I sit up, hearing the urgency in his voice. "I need to complete my life's work before it is too late."

Father wants to tell his story so his family can remember him when he is gone. Father hopes to achieve immortality through his writing, not for the sake of fame or fortune, but to leave behind the legacy of his life for his children and his children's children.

I weigh the enormity of his proposition. It would be a formidable undertaking. I am uncertain whether I have what it takes as a writer to help my father pen his final swan song. Yet I am moved that my father believes in me enough to trust me with this final creative work.

"Yes, of course I will help you. It would be an honor."

"Kagan, you must go on living. We cannot prevent what is going to happen to me. You have your whole life ahead of you."

"Dad, I want you to be around when I get married. I want you to be there when my children are born. I can't imagine life without you."

"I have had a good sixty-nine years. I have lived a full life. But I am not giving up yet. We can't afford to postpone our lives any longer. No use lying in bed feeling depressed. Come on. Get out of bed. It's a beautiful day. Let's go into the garden."

Father unlatches the gate to our garden. We have two pear trees, an apple tree, a plum tree, a cherry tree and a grape vine in our garden. He inspects the flower buds appearing on the fruit trees, the first sign of spring in the air. Brushing aside overhanging branches and spider webs, we discover that the garden is overgrown with weeds.

"The garden is a mess," my father says, "Let's get to work!"

Father wastes no time and fetches the gardening tools out of the shed. We spend the rest of the afternoon trimming the branches and pulling weeds.

After a hard day's work, he pats me on the back. "Tomorrow we'll buy seeds and plant some flowers."

Bright and early the next morning, he wakes me to go grocery shopping. I select apples and oranges from the fruit stands outside Donald's Market, our local Chinese grocery store. Father stops me from putting apples and oranges into the basket.

"I'm bored with eating apples and oranges all the time. Let's buy peaches, plums, apricots, grapes and strawberries. I want to eat more decadent fruits. Let's treat ourselves, spoil ourselves a little."

Next, we stop off at Figaro's Garden, a nursery where all manner of flora can be bought. We enter intending to buy some flower seeds and leave carrying a few potted plants and flowers as well. Returning home, father plants the seeds in fertile soil. As he waters the seeds he has sown, he coaxes them to grow:

"Grow my little lovelies. Grow into beautiful flowers so our garden will be glorious for summer parties."

Having worked up an appetite, father uses the blender to make a healthy fruit smoothie with a dollop of yogurt and a spoonful of honey. Famished, I inhale my breakfast like a starving man.

"You eat like a prisoner guarding your food from other inmates," observes father. "Slow down. How do you even taste your food if you eat so quickly? Take your time and enjoy your food."

I eat slower, feeling slightly embarrassed.

"That's better. Savor every morsel and it will make you immortal."

After breakfast, father walks from room to room and plans to improve our home.

"Let us paint the walls and lay new carpet on the floor. I want to renovate the bathroom and kitchen as well. This is our family home. Let's make this a house we can be proud of."

That same day, we go to Home Depot to buy paint, select carpet and look at new kitchen and bathroom designs for the apartments.

Father is a man of action. His motto is: "Those who do, dare. Those who fear, fail." Father looks ahead to the future. Not the attitude of a man facing death. Instead, he is drunk on the rage of being alive.

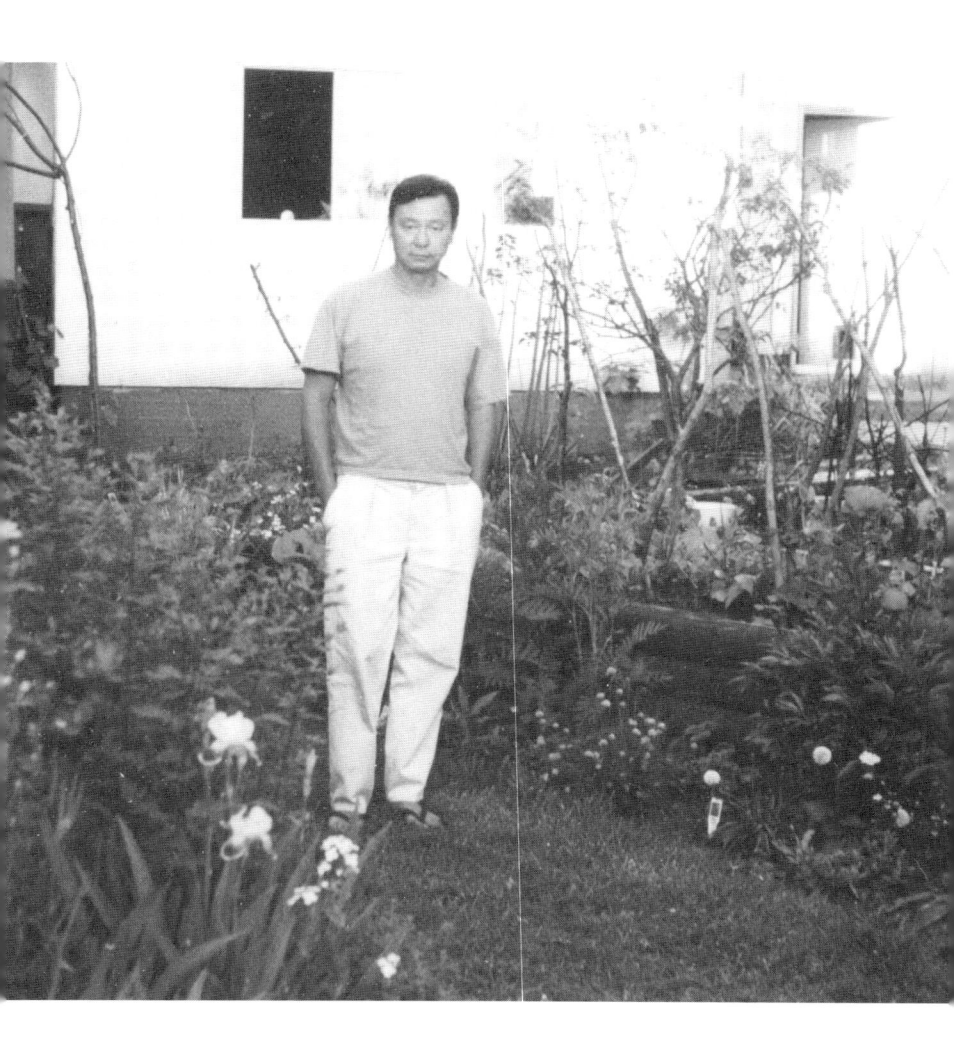

THE FIRST DAY BACK

The day father was released from hospital after the cancer operation, he was relieved and overjoyed to hear that he did not need chemotherapy. His cancer was in remission.

The doctor instructed him to rest and take it easy. The family was poised, ready for a period of convalescence in which he would have to be cared for and attended to.

We rented a mechanized bed that would make it easier for him to sit up and get out of bed. We got him a walker in case he needed assistance getting around. We got a commode in case he had difficulty getting to the toilet.

We expected father's recovery to be a slow and patient process. But the minute he got back from the hospital, he was already walking unassisted, cooking, cleaning and gardening. On the first day back he decided he wanted to get fit and started an exercise regime. He boasted that he did more than a hundred sit-ups and pushups.

In the evening, father went for a jog around Trout Lake Park. My father, a man of seventy with Parkinson's disease ran around the park, legs stiff, muscles aching, lungs inflating and deflating like two balloons, working up a sweat giving the young joggers a run for their money.

At the end of the day we gave up trying to restrain him. Father's zest for life is an inspiration to us all. When he gets going, there is no stopping him. Way to go Dad!

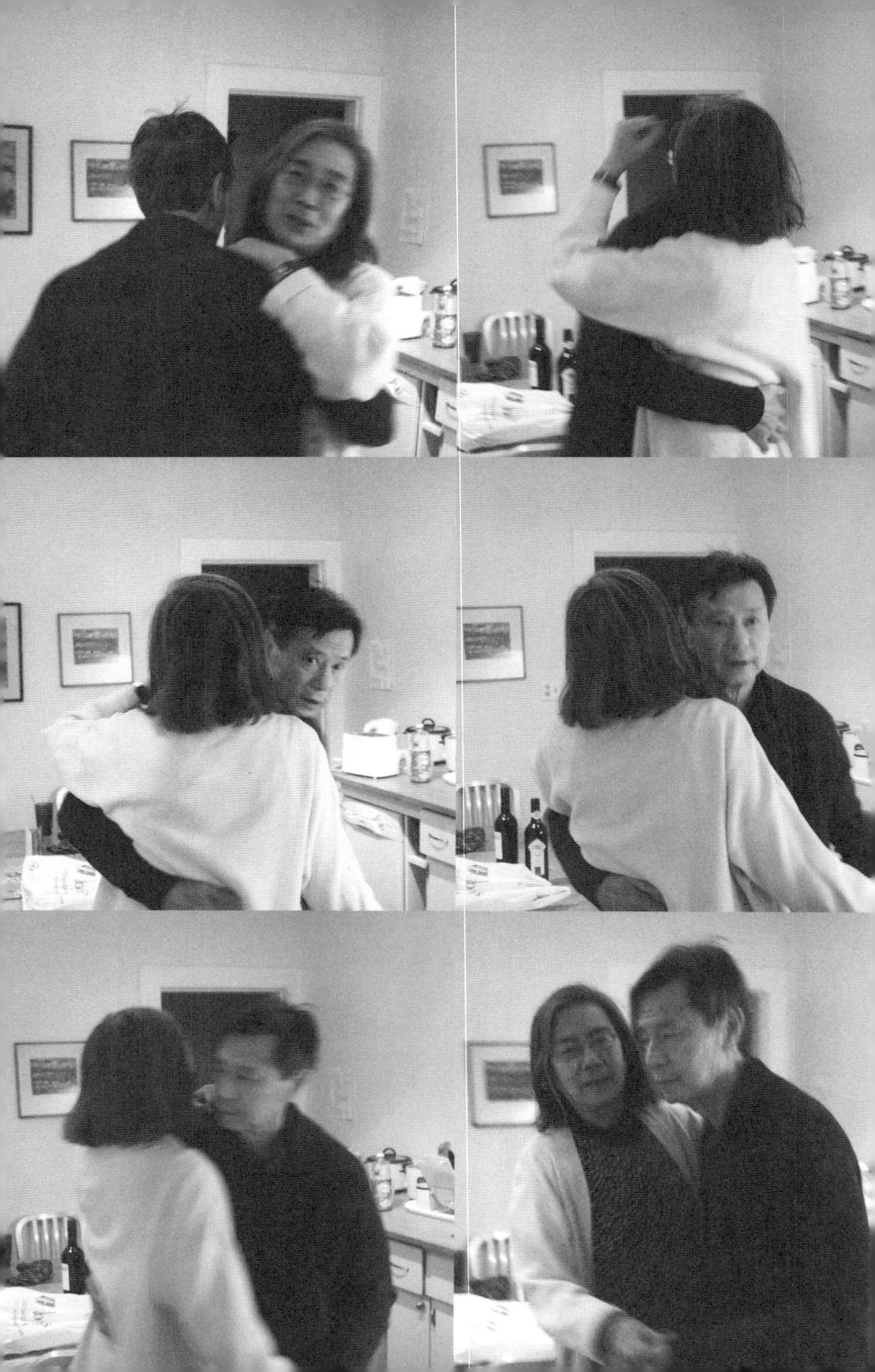

MY SWEET EMBRACEABLE YOU

It almost didn't happen. I didn't want to go, wasn't in the mood, but Mum kept haranguing me, and wouldn't let me be a spoilsport. Finally I agreed. We bundled up, braved the rain and made our way to the Legion to go swing dancing on a Saturday night. I lugged the wheelchair up two flights of stairs while Mum helped Dad climb up the precarious steps to the dance hall.

I remember the song by the big band, the sweet melody, that sentimental refrain by Ira and George Gershwin.

"Embrace me,
My sweet embraceable you.
Embrace me,
My irreplaceable you.
Just to look at you
My heart grows tipsy in me.
You and you alone
Bring out the gypsy in me."

Dad and Mum were the most beautiful couple on the dance floor that night. Beautiful because they were the most loving couple of all. The youngsters had fancier dance moves but no one moved more gracefully or lovely than the two of them. That night Dad and Mum recaptured the romance of their relationship. It was magic! I felt so lucky to have been there to witness both of my parents become young again, the years sloughing off their skin like the bark of a Eucalyptus tree, to reveal both of them young, healthy and happy again.

Dad was a terrific dancer, and so was Mum. Dad's Parkinson's was gone. Cured! Mum's anxieties just melted away. We all felt it. How special that moment was. Everyone else just disappeared in the dance hall leaving both of them alone drifting away amidst the Milky Way. Two innocent sweethearts, unrepentant romantic fools unabashed about the affection and love they felt for each other.

"Sweet," my parents have always called each other that all their lives. "My Sweet," a beautiful term of endearment. When I was young I mistook what they were saying for "sweat"; but how appropriate, the sweet sweat of tears of joy mingling with tears of sorrow, the bittersweet brewery of love distilled over a lifetime.

That night Mum was Dad's gal. Dad was Mum's fella. Both of them were stellar, spectacular! That was the last time I would ever see my parents dance together. A few days later Mum almost died of a vascular aneurism. A week later Dad suffered a relapse of aspiration pneumonia. Two months later he passed away. I will never see my parents dance again. And to think I did not want to go. Now I no longer put things off, waiting for tomorrow when today may never come again. Whenever I miss Dad and feel sad, I hold onto that burning vision of him and Mum slow dancing at the Legion. Hear the big band playing that bittersweet refrain:

"I love all
The many charms about you.
Above all
I want my arms about you.
Don't be naughty baby,
Come to Papa
Come to Papa do
My sweet embraceable you."

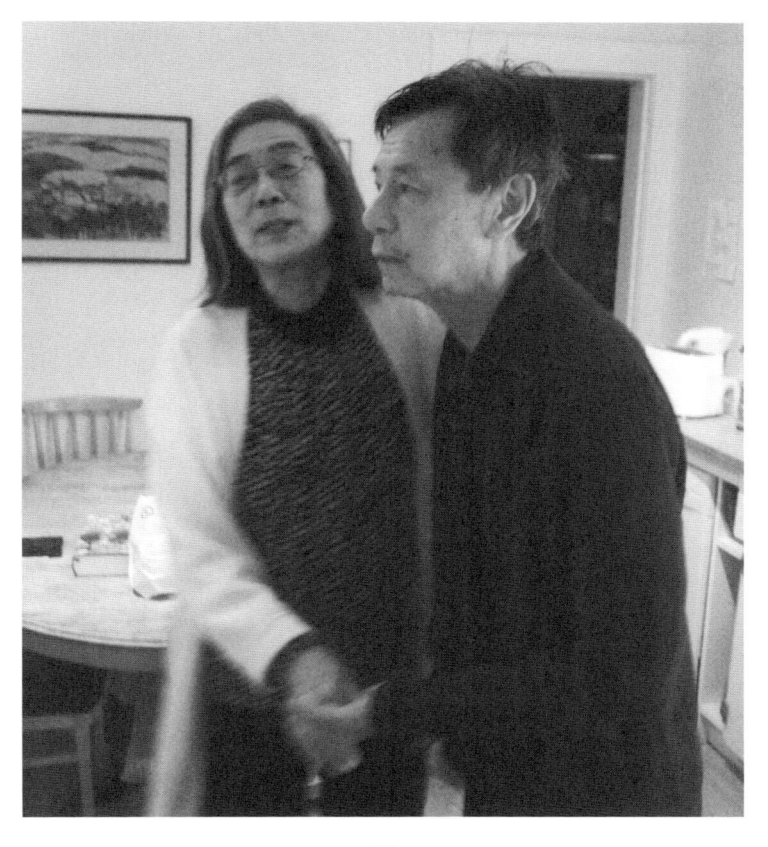

THE GOOD FIGHT

Every night at bedtime, just as my father is about to fall asleep, he hallucinates that my mother steals out under the cloak of darkness to go frolicking at jovial parties without him. Perhaps he fears she may be having affairs, suspecting rendezvous with imaginary lovers behind his back.

I find it amusing that my father dreams my mother has a jolly good time at night, when in fact she is dead asleep, exhausted from the demands of care-taking and the unrelenting catastrophes that seem to inundate her life.

My father has never accepted the limitations imposed upon him by Parkinson's disease. I admire his fighting spirit, his refusal to succumb to depression and give up on life. He has never felt sorry for himself. Instead he is determined to live life on his own terms despite his illness.

He suffers from fainting spells, brought on by dangerously low blood pressure. His fainting spells are frightening. He blacks out and falls the way a tree falls in a forest; the whole weight of his body comes crashing down. He has had numerous stitches on his head and once even broke his arm. Walking with a cane makes no difference. The fainting spells are so frequent, as many as twelve a day, that his doctor advises him to use a wheelchair. But my father refuses to accept this disability, choosing instead to risk the falls.

When my father gets frustrated and angry, he storms out of the house in a temper tantrum, refusing to tell us where he is going. He refuses to listen to his family's attempts to reason with him, seeing our concern for his risk-taking behaviour as an unacceptable restriction of his freedom. He blackmails us emotionally, feeling the only way he can make his family care is to make us worry for his safety, so he puts himself in harms way, exerting his independence in the only way he knows: self-destructively.

"I would rather die than listen to you!"

Invariably he ends up falling and injuring himself. Kind passersby will call the ambulance and they will take him to the emergency ward of the hospital. Meanwhile we sit and wait anxiously by the phone for the fateful call. We have become so accustomed to the routine that we simply wait for the call from the hospital, praying he is safe and has not come to a bad end, fearful that he might get run over by a vehicle while crossing the road.

I have always been afraid of my father dying. Little did I suspect that my mother would be the first one in our family to be courted by death. One morning, Mum collapses on the floor of her bedroom experiencing excruciating spasms of pain in her abdomen and back. I summon an ambulance, which arrives within minutes. When the ambulance attendants take Mum away, she insists they take Dad along because he is sick with pneumonia. Even at the brink of death, she thinks of him first. If this is not evidence of true love, I do not know what is.

I admit Dad to Saint Paul's Hospital's emergency ward at the same time as Mum. Dad is so worried about Mum that he refuses to be treated for pneumonia. More concerned about his wife's wellbeing, he checks himself out of the emergency ward against the doctor's advice. The doctor informs him that his wife is in critical condition. The doctors diagnose Mum with a vascular aneurism, a rupture in her aorta. Nine out of ten patients who undergo surgery for this condition die. Due to the seriousness of her condition, the surgeons decide to operate immediately.

In the waiting room, I try to contemplate the inconceivable. "Your mother might not survive," cautions Dad. "We must brace ourselves for whatever is going to happen."

The operation takes six hours. An eternity. Finally, a nurse informs us: "Your wife survived the operation. Thank goodness! She is lucky to be alive."

Later that night, I help my father change for bed. I tuck him into bed just as he had done so for me when I was a child. I enjoy the ritual, this slow intimate dance between father and son.

"Dad, we nearly lost Mum today. We're lucky to still have her with us. She has devoted her life to take care of you. She's been a real trouper and has done everything she possibly can to make your life comfortable. But the stress of looking after you is so great it nearly killed her. We have to face the fact that she can no longer look after you anymore. We've been putting this off for as long as possible but I believe it is time to explore the option of a nursing home. I know you don't like the idea of being separated from the family but the truth is, even with the homecare workers coming seven days a week, we still can't manage to look after you."

"I knew this day would come sooner or later," he replies lucidly. "I've seen some of the nursing homes. They're not so bad," he says, unconvincingly. "I admit I'm not keen about the idea but I will simply have to learn to adapt."

Nearly losing his wife has sobered him up to reality. I am moved by how he has chosen to accept his fate with grace and dignity.

"We will come to visit you every day. We'll take you out for excursions and bring your favourite meals."

"I am lucky to have a son like you."

"I love you Dad. You and Mum are my best friends."

"I love you too."

He purses his lips. We kiss goodnight. Even at forty years old, a grown man kissing his father goodnight, pausing to look back at him sink into sleep before turning out the light.

The next day, Dad and I visit Mum at the Intensive Care Unit. The nurse leads us to her bed. Hooked up to a battery of machines, Mum is frail and weak. Dad sidles up to her and holds her hand.

"Are you upset with me?"

A strained look appears on her brow. "It's always about you and how you feel! Please let me rest. I almost died. Leave me in peace!"

I wheel Dad away in his wheelchair, creating a buffer between him and Mum so she can recover.

Later that afternoon, we eat lunch in silence at a delicatessen near the hospital.

In the middle of the meal, father suddenly protests: "I am not going to a nursing home. All of you will abandon me. I have nothing in common with those old people. I will waste away and die alone there. I refuse to go and that's final!"

"Dad, we've discussed this before. We'll find you a nice nursing home. We have no choice."

"I simply refuse to go. I will move out and get an apartment of my own."

"Who will take care of you?"

"I can take care of myself. I can get one of those homecare workers to take care of me."

"The homecare workers come for only five hours a day. You need round the clock care. Who is willing to dedicate all the days of their life to take care of you the way Mum did?"

My father broods in silence. I am unable to break the deadlock between us. On the way back to the hospital, father accuses me of neglecting mother.

"You claim the reason she almost died is because of the stress of looking after me. What about the stress of looking after you? Night after night she complains that she never knows whether you're coming home to eat dinner."

"The reason why I don't come home for dinner is because I can't stand the two of you fighting all the time."

"Maybe you are the one who drove her over the edge!"

That's the final straw. In a rush of anger, I shove his wheelchair and let go of the handles, shouting: "Asshole!"

I derive perverse satisfaction from my outburst, but the next moment I am swamped with guilt, regretting my impulsive action. I chase after the runaway wheelchair and manage to grab hold of the handles before it veers towards traffic.

"Trying to kill your own father! Let me go! Get out of my way! Wait till your mother hears about this!" he protests.

He wheels himself through the hospital entrance, manages somehow to open the door and wheels himself down the corridor, swearing and ranting angrily at me, heading in the direction of my mother's ward. I wonder how my father is going to figure out how to get to her ward on his own with his poor sense of direction. But father lets no one get in his way when he is in a rage. By the time I catch up with him, it is too late. I find my weary mother listening to my father's complaints. In total exasperation she pleads:

"Sweet, please! I can't hear this. I need to rest. Please leave me alone. Don't come to see me if you are going to behave like this."

Father sags in total defeat. I wheel him out of the hospital, away from her.

Outside the hospital, I hail a taxi to take us home. Dad demands: "Give me my keys and bank card! I'm going off on my own."

I refuse to comply with his request. Once, after an argument with Mum, Dad got on an airplane and flew off to Saint John's, Newfoundland on his own and went on a spending spree with his credit card. Learning from precedent, I am not about to let history repeat itself. Over my dead body.

Back home, the situation gets worse. I pay the taxi driver and bring Dad into the house. "Give me the keys and bank card now!" I ignore him and lock the front gate behind me to prevent him from leaving the house. I do not want to contend with another scenario where my father storms off on his own, putting himself in harm's way. Dad berates me as I retreat and lock myself in Mum's bedroom for safety from his verbal abuse. He bangs on the door, demanding I give him his money and house keys. After a while, Dad stops banging on the door. I open the door and check to see if the coast is clear. No sign of Dad. The apartment is empty. I find Dad has rooted through the tool closet and used a hammer to smash a hole in the wooden fence of the house, creating a gap through which he made his escape.

 I sit up all day until late night when I receive a phone call. I answer, expecting to hear from the hospital. To my surprise, I hear the voice of Uncle Chin Nan informing me Dad is safe with him. Apparently he had called my uncle who promptly came and fetched him. Dad had been enjoying Auntie Seok Imm's delicious Peranakan home cooking, all the while unloading his troubles upon them, ranting and raving about how his family had ganged up on him. I was upset that my uncle had waited all this time, making me worry unnecessarily all night long about the safety of my father.

 Concerned about Dad's deteriorating health, Uncle Chin Nan checks him into hospital for observation. In the following weeks, during Mum's absence, Dad's spark diminishes. Against the doctor's advice, he checked himself out of the hospital and consequently suffers a serious relapse of pneumonia and is admitted to the Saint Paul's Hospital's geriatric ward.

 My father suffers from aspiration pneumonia. When he eats or drinks, he has difficulty swallowing and the food and liquid goes down the wrong passage into his lungs. I follow the doctor's advice by feeding my father pureed food that is easier to swallow. He protests when I feed him applesauce with a plastic spoon.

"Let's go to a restaurant. I want real food. Not this baby food."

He ignores the doctor's warning and chooses to eat solid food at risk. Father refuses to deprive himself of one of the last pleasures he has left: good food. An average person would have difficulty recovering from one bout of pneumonia. In the past three years he has survived twelve bouts of aspiration pneumonia. Father's spirit is strong although his body is weak. He is determined to stay alive against all odds.

My brother Kajin flies back home from Toronto to help take care of Mum and Dad and support the family during this crisis. Kajin and I consult with the doctors, nurses and social workers. We are informed that Dad has been rebelling against the hospital staff, nurses and doctors because he is being held under the Mental Health Act. In the doctor's opinion, my father poses a danger to himself and needs to be detained in the hospital against his will for his own good. He fights with all his might he has lost insight. He won't listen to reason and sees our concern for him as an attempt to control his life. But, angered and stubborn beyond reason, believing there is a conspiracy against him, he is fighting the wrong fight, pitting himself against those who are trying to help him.

Dad wants to get out of bed. He attempts to climb over the railings of the hospital bed. He ends up landing hard on the floor, hurting his head. Two nurses attempt to tie his hands to his bed railings to prevent him from climbing out of bed again.

"Let me go! It's my right to go home!" Dad wrestles with the nurses. He injures one so badly she has bruises, resulting in him being sedated.

Dad wants to get out of hospital. He wants to go home. The hope of going home is the only reason keeping him alive. But home is no longer an option, even for us. Mum might have to move into a seniors' home. The family will have to sell the house. Kajin and I will have to leave our beloved Commercial Drive neighbourhood where we have lived for sixteen years. Major upheaval lies ahead in our lives and it is not going to be easy for any of us.

Kajin is keeping vigil over Dad. He shares a room with six other patients. The smell of old people suffering from incontinence fills the air; a mixture of urine and excrement makes my brother sick to the stomach. Kajin draws the curtain around my father's bed for privacy.

"Get me out of here! This place is for old people," my father begs. "I don't want to die here! I want to go home!"

"Sorry Dad. That is not possible. Mum can no longer take care of you." Kajin tries to reason with him. "Neither can we. Your health has deteriorated so badly we can't manage even with help from home care workers seven days a week. Please reconsider the option of a nursing home."

"I will die there, waste away and be forgotten. All of you will abandon me."

Visiting hours are over. My father waving his cane in protest, follows Kajin into the corridor, berating him as he walks towards the exit.

"Get me out of here! I don't want to die here! Obey your father! Are you going to force me to stay here in this hospital against my will? What kind of a son abandons his own father? Oh I give up! What's the use?"

Hearing the dejection in his voice, Kajin's heart sinks.

"Sorry Dad I can't…" He exits the door. It locks behind him, shutting our father in.

My father's health takes a turn for the worse. I make a request to the head nurse whether he can be moved to a private room because one of his roommates keeps babbling, "Oh, I am in pain. My arse hurts!" over and over again, driving my father insane. The nurse is kind and grants my request. My father's bed is wheeled into a single room with a nice view of the West End. Through the window Christmas lights blink in the pattern of a star, a beacon of hope pulsating into the heart of the dreary winter night.

My father looks shrunken, a mere ghost of the man he once was. He is feeble and weak from fighting all week. Now all the fight is gone out of him. I do not know which is worse, him fighting the forces he perceives stand in the way of his freedom, or the fear he will stop fighting and give up altogether, surrender and let depression overcome him.

"How is my father doing?" I ask the head nurse. "Is he going to pull through?"

"Pneumonia is known as "the Old Man's Friend." To be frank, your father is dying of old age. The next twenty-four to forty-eight hours are critical. I advise you to notify his close relatives. If you have anything to say to him, now is the time to say goodbye."

I call my brothers Kasan and Kakim and inform them of the situation. "This is his third bout of pneumonia since he arrived in hospital. The disease has infected his kidneys; the toxins have affected his mental faculty. He's delirious and has been delusional since the weekend. He goes in and out of lucidity. He might not recognize anyone." I tell them to come as soon as possible if they can. Kakim, my youngest brother, leaves work in Montreal and flies over to Vancouver to see Dad. He risks losing his new job where he is on probation. Kasan, my eldest brother who lives in England, is torn, wondering whether he can spare the time to get away to see Dad who may not even recognize him.

Kajin, Kakim and I take turns keeping vigil over Dad, feeding him his favourite food, reading him his own poems. He claps his hands in delight: "Good poem! Good poem!" His mind is reverting to a child-like state. During the night he calls for his childhood servants and deceased relatives, talking to them as if they are present in the room.

At Saint Paul's Hospital's geriatric ward sitting by my father's bedside, I watch him drift in and out of consciousness, unable to speak except for indecipherable mumbles, driven mad by loneliness and the loss of the life he once knew, feeling abandoned by his family, isolated and alone in this cold ward where people come to die.

I read to father a Dylan Thomas poem.

"Do not go gentle into that good night,
Old age should burn and rave at close of day;
Rage, rage against the dying of the light.

And you, my father, there on the sad height,
Curse, bless, me now with your fierce tears, I pray.
Do not go gentle into that good night.
Rage, rage against the dying of the light."

His breathing is laboured. He struggles to breathe through plastic tubes stuck up his nostrils. He is being fed by saline solution dripping into a tube in his arm from an IV. Having lost his appetite and not eaten for a week, he has lost a lot of weight and looks thin and skeletal. I look into the dim spark of my father's eyes, searching for signs of life.

"Dad, do you recognize me? Squeeze my hand if you know who I am."

I clutch his hand. He squeezes. His grip is weak, like a little child's.

"Please forgive me Dad. I'm sorry. I didn't mean to hurt you. I love you so much. You weren't trying to be difficult. You were just scared to be separated from your family."

Tears fill his eyes.

"You are the best friend I have ever had," I confess. "I don't know how I am going to go on without you."

Under his blanket, I massage my father's calf and thigh muscles. They hang limp and soft. His muscle tone is gone from being bedridden for weeks. His eyes swim in delirium, caught in the hallucinatory state between sleep and wakefulness.

"Mum loves you more than you will ever know. If you have any doubts about her loyalty, remember this. Every night when you think she is stealing out of the house to go partying, she is in fact leaving the house, not to escape or abandon you, but instead to prepare a party, the greatest surprise party in your honour."

Consoling him, I become the Dreamweaver, spinning happy hallucinations for my father.

"Get strong Dad. Keep up the good fight. Fight the right fight for the right reasons. Fight to live. Above all, fight to love."

I kiss him on his forehead.

"I know you don't believe in God or don't want to believe in God. Instead believe in your family. Believe that we love you. We will never leave you. We will do anything for you. We are all here waiting for you. Hiding in the dark. Waiting for you to get well, wake up, open your eyes and then to spring the surprise, cheering: "It is your forty-eighth wedding anniversary!" Mum and you celebrating together your golden honeymoon in the bosom of your family. Do not worry. You are not alone. We are here waiting to take you home."

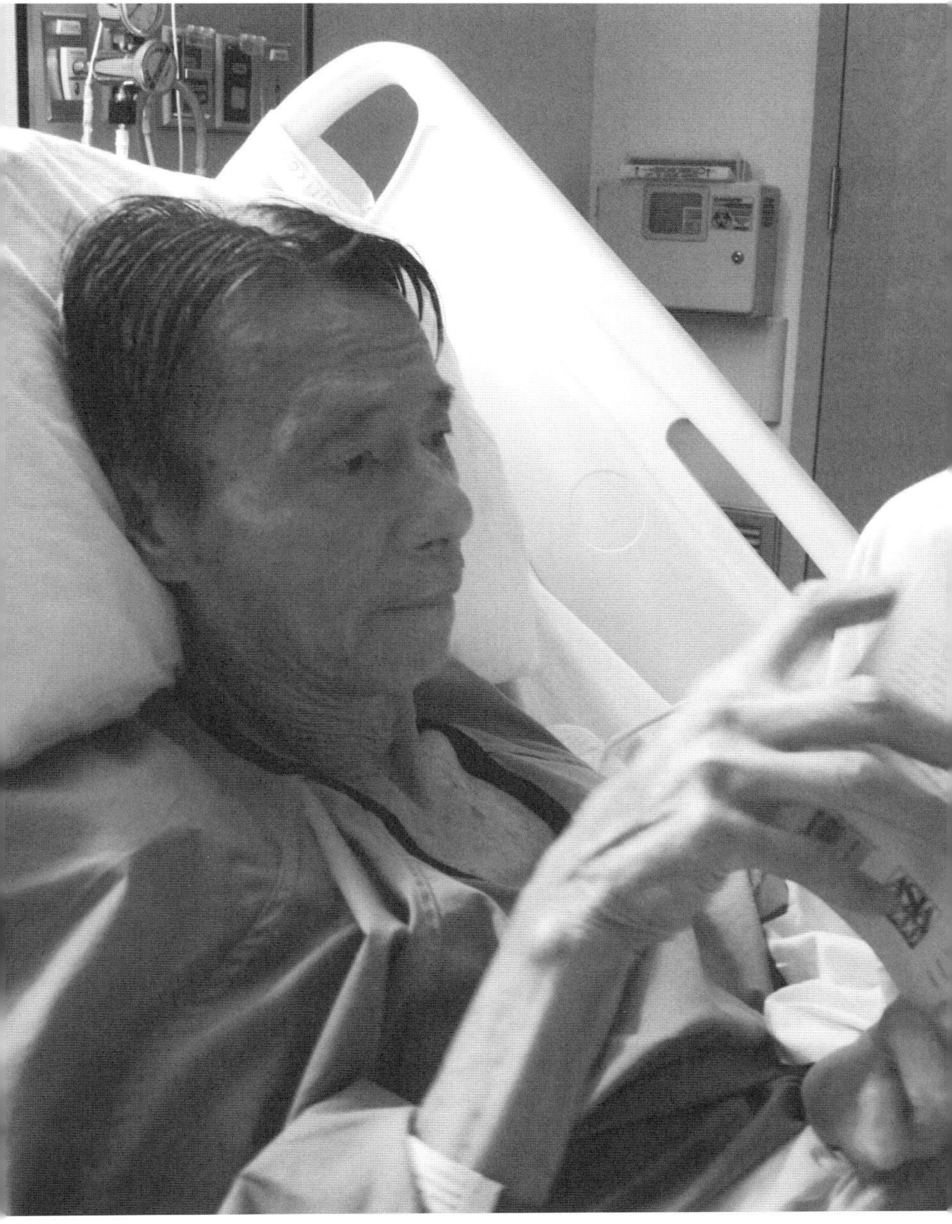

WALKING AMONGST GHOSTS

My father walks amongst ghosts. Returning home late one night, he tells me he see phantoms in the shadows. He points into the darkness.

"Why is that man sitting on the curb?"

All I see is a black garbage bag and recycling bin left by the curbside waiting to be picked up by the garbage truck the next morning.

He points to a tree. "Look! There is a man sitting on the tree branch!"

I look up at the branches of the tree and half expect to see the Cheshire cat grin at me. All I see is the smile of the crescent moon.

"Dad, there is no one there. Your mind is playing tricks on you."

Back home, father undresses for bed. I help him pee into the piss pot. After he is done, I help him put on his diapers. I lay out a dry pad on his bed and newspaper on the floor in case he wets himself. The indignity of old age, being treated like a baby. Tucking him under the covers, father points his finger, counting out loud.

"One. Two. Three. Four. Five. Six…"

"What are you doing Dad?"

"I am counting the number of people in the room."

I am the only person in the bedroom. A shiver runs up my spine, unnerved by the thought there are people in our presence I cannot see. Father sees things no one else can.

On another occasion, father sits in the living room and peers out the window on a sunny day. He tells me he sees a group of English ladies and gentlemen, dressed in white, playing badminton in our garden, laughing and frolicking about in great merriment.

"Can't you see them? They are making a loud racket."

"Dad, no one is in the garden."

His visitations by invisible folk are so life-like, so real to him and have become so frequent that I have come to believe ghosts visit my father. In the final days of his life, father walks between the shadows of the living and the dead. He has one foot in this world and the other foot in the afterlife.

Father spends so much time in the world of ghosts that eventually his turn comes to cross over. Father lies in a hospital bed. He complains about the noise from the Chinese opera troupe playing next door. The ward is silent except for the beep of the electro cardiogram machine.

Father's final hallucination is as follows: he tells me that he is crossing a bridge with his fellow poets to go a poetry reading. He tells me the poetry is inspiring, the food marvelous and the wine free flowing. Father is so frail; death is just a whisper away. His deceased poet friends wait patiently for my father. The invisible ghosts gather around to keep him company. Hearing them beckon him, he crosses the bridge to join their ranks. Standing on the bridge, he hesitates a moment, turns to look back one last time and waves goodbye. Like a Brahmin he ventures forth to become a holy man walking the final road to the Holy Land. The great poets welcome him at the gates of heaven. He is reunited with Gerry Gilbert, Billy Little, Al Pitman and Charles Watts. They kick up a holy ruckus loud enough to wake God and scare the Devil.

Tears well up in his eyes.

His last breath a sigh.

Goodbye.

He's going.

He's going.

He's gone.

He's gone to the other side of dawn.

The tide recedes.

Father's soul has departed its corporeal shell.

His eyes are open, so life-like

but the spark within has vanished.

I kiss him on the forehead and then on the lips.

Cold to the touch

I recoil.

I sit by father's bedside

and read him poems.

I keep vigil

all night till the dawn

singing songs to guide his soul to the light.

He is gone,

but his presence still remains.

A vibrating light

hovers in the room.

Death cannot eclipse his soul.

Father haunts me as a ghost,
keeps me company
during my lonely days without him.
Father, will you be my voice of hope
at times when I can't cope?
When I am scared,
father comforts me in dreams.
He accompanies me arm in arm
down the spiral staircase into darkness.
He is my constant companion.
Not even death can separate us.
We wander through the Dark Forest of the Night,
our path lit by the lantern light of our souls.

Death is not the end.
We all live in an Open House with many rooms.
When someone dies, they merely leave this room
and enter another one.
We can no longer see them
but they still live in the same house.
When my time comes to cross over,
I will be reunited with my father.
Keep the porch light on Dad.
Wait for me.
I will be home to stay with you
for the rest of my living and undying days.

GOD IS DEAD

After years of serving him,
tending to his every whim and desire,
I saw him lying there
still in the shadow of death,
cold as stone.
Instead of the ground opening up
and swallowing him,
the sky grew heavy
and came crashing down.

Vancouver, 2010

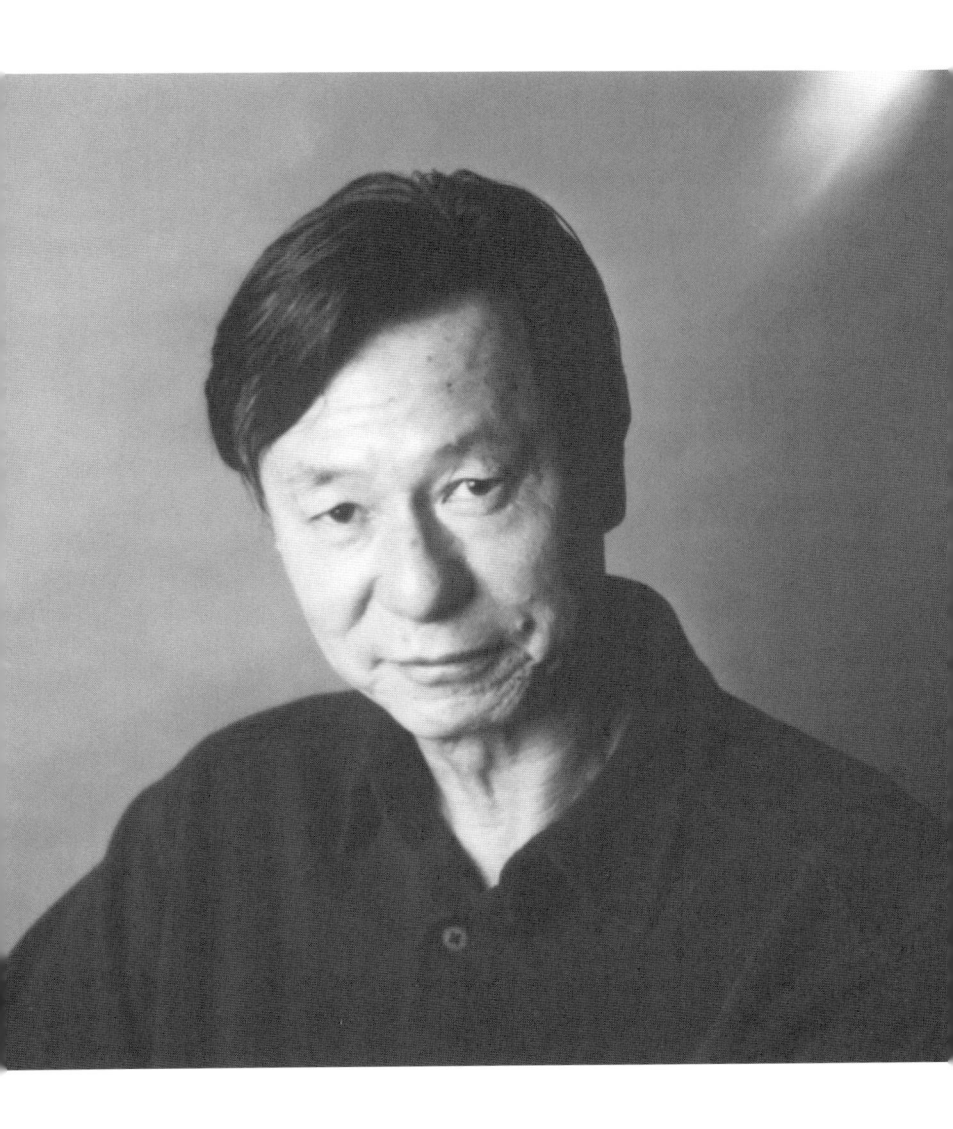

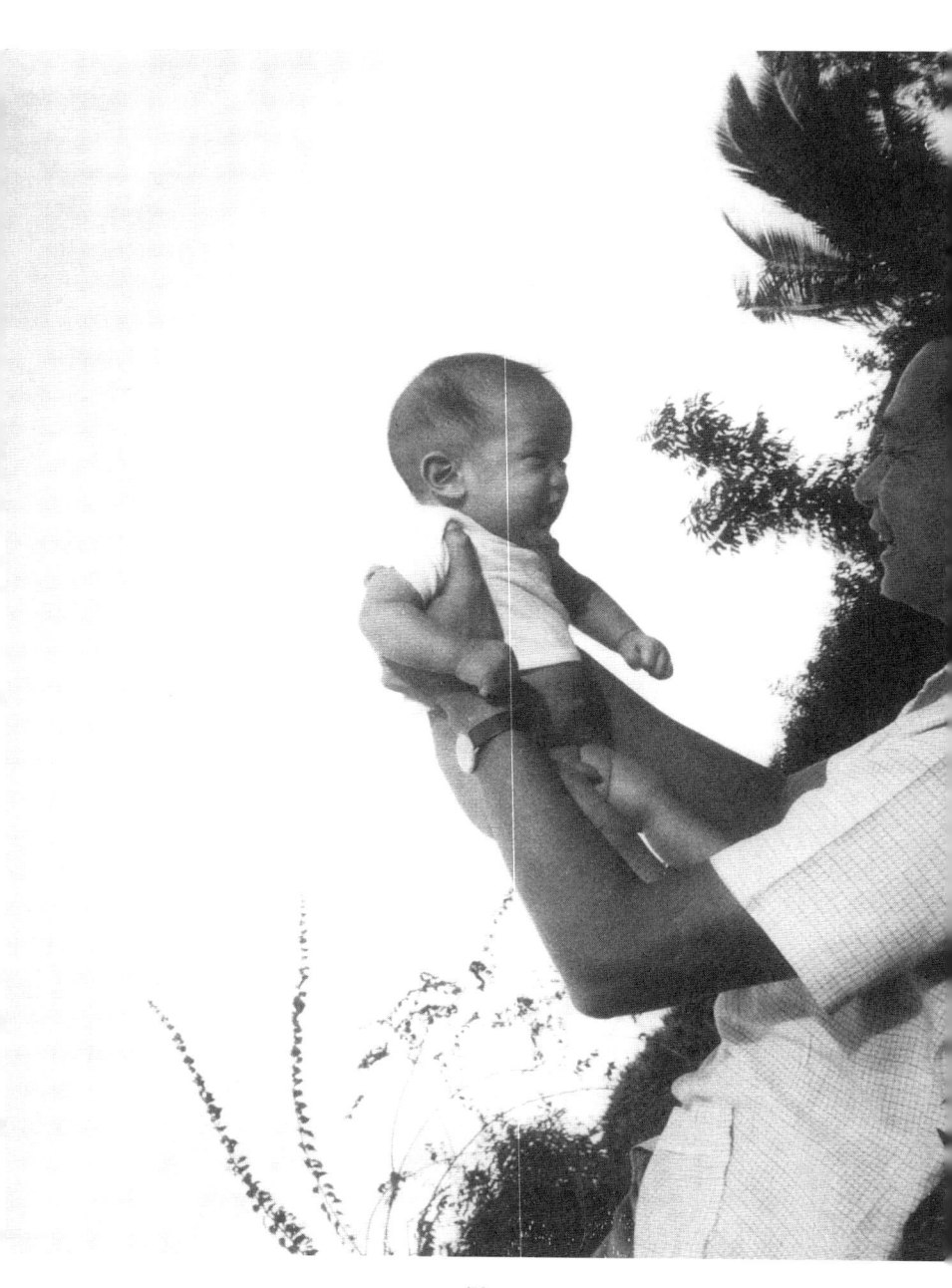

SNAPSHOT

My father holds a baby
with his strong arms up to the sky.
My father
larger than life
lies on the grass
defying gravity itself
the earth pressed vertically against his back.
A proud father
unabashed about his love for his child.
He holds me up to the sky
high above the trees.
I squeal as he presents me to God.
"Creator, bless my beloved son
whom I love more than life itself.
Protect him. Keep him safe
for the rest of his living and undying days."
Father held me with his strong arms
all my life until the day he died.
Reluctantly father let go
handing me to God.

Vancouver, 2010

A STRONG FRONT

She had been holding up quite well so far considering the circumstances. After the surgery, the doctor told her nine out of ten patients with her condition do not survive. She was lucky to be alive. A week after her attack, her husband was admitted into the same hospital for aspiration pneumonia. She was on the tenth floor and he a floor below on the ninth. She was worried he would defy the doctors and nurses and storm the ward to see her.

When she was discharged she checked into a hotel a block away from the hospital. She slept for two weeks, too weak to summon up the strength and energy to visit him. Meanwhile he languished in her absence.

When she finally recovered sufficiently to visit him, she was horrified at how thin and gaunt he was. She was shocked at how quickly he had deteriorated in her absence, as if without her he simply could not survive and had wasted away. He was all skin and bones and looked like an Auschwitz victim. He was hallucinating, delusional, and had reverted to speaking in Hokkien, his mother tongue. He called out to his servant who had long since died:

"Ah Siew Chia, bite off my hand! BITE OFF MY HAND!"

He struggled, hitting his arm violently as if an invisible dog was biting his hand and he was trying to shake loose of its jaws. His family tried to restrain him from hurting himself. It took three of them to hold him down. They were surprised how strong he still was. He spoke with a Malaysian accent and sounded eerily like his dead father. It was as if he had returned to a child-like state, as if nearing death he was drinking from the same river of his childhood, death and birth coming full circle. The circle of life, a serpent swallowing its own tail; in the end one returns to where one began.

She started visiting him more frequently as her strength returned. Day by day she saw him slip away into the ether, one foot already in the next world. She would spend the day with him, taking shifts with her sons, keeping vigil over her dying husband. When he slept, she would look out the window. Amidst the tall red brick buildings of the hospital, there was a tiny house, more a little cabin, set in a small courtyard amidst an Oriental bamboo grove. It was strange to see this haven of peace and tranquility amidst the domineering larger buildings. She took comfort in this sanctuary.

When she received the phone call from her son, - "Come quickly, Dad's body is shutting down. He is slipping away," she did not realize the true urgency of the message. She stopped off at a grocery store to buy food for dinner, then made her way to the hospital, but she entered the wrong entrance. By the time she got to his room, she had missed him by a few precious minutes. If only she had not stopped for groceries. If only she had taken the right entrance. She cried into his chest, stroking his hair, grief stricken that she did not have a chance to say goodbye. His eyes were still open, so life-like but the spark within was gone. His flesh was cold to the touch.

Well-meaning friends and relatives assailed her, offering love and support, but she found it hard to be with people. She held up a strong front, as she had done all her life and kept herself busy. She was surprised in the weeks after he died she had not cried. All that changed one day when she returned to the hospital for a routine checkup. Looking out the window she saw the little cabin amidst the concrete jungle. Reminded of her husband, she burst into tears, sobbing uncontrollably. She felt he now dwelled in the solace of that little sanctuary amidst the tall gleaming headstones in heaven.

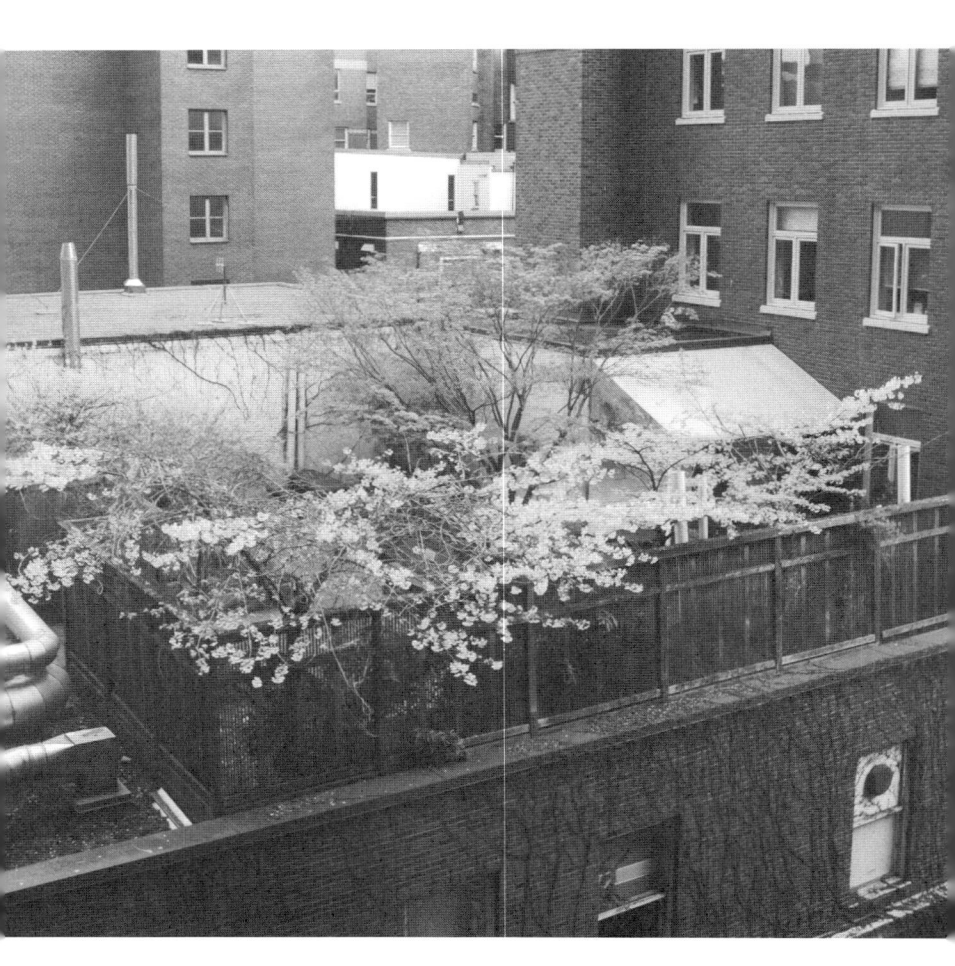

BEEPER

The son was tidying up his parents' apartment, packing away his father's belongings after the wake, preparing for his mother's return home from the hotel, a life without her husband. Their family had emigrated and moved several times in his short life, so much so he had become accustomed to living out of boxes. Even so, this was the hardest packing job he ever had to do, packing his father's belongings, sorting what to keep, what to give away and what to throw out. He felt reluctant to get rid of his father's belongings, even insignificant junk.

Every item reminded him of his father. His father's many toothpicks, found scattered along kitchen counters and on the floor made him nostalgic. What to do with the urine catheters? He decided he would donate them to the Home Respite Center where his father resided when his mother needed a break from care-taking. He decided to pocket his father's comb, noticing a few strands of hair stuck in its teeth.

Suddenly, out of the blue, he heard a beeping sound. Beep beep beep... He wandered throughout the apartment trying to locate its source. Where was it coming from? Beep beep beep... He followed the sound and finally traced it to a cardboard box. He rummaged through its contents and found the beeper. A white plastic double-A battery-operated digital timer which had been used to remind his father to take his medication every three hours, six times a day. Doses at 7 am, 10 am, 1 pm, 4 pm, 7 pm and finally ending at 10 pm.

It had been a source of great anxiety and stress to the family keeping track of when to remind and dispense meds to his father. Also in the cardboard box was a satchel with his father's medications and several plastic pill dispensers. The countless years, months, weeks, days, hours, minutes and seconds spent worrying about him absentmindedly misplacing or losing his pill dispensers drove his family to distraction. He had to take an endless battery of pills religiously several times a day for his Parkinson's, otherwise his body would stiffen and a whole horrific onslaught of side-effects would assail him. His father took this cruel communion, swallowing pill after pill every day for the last fifteen years. It drove him crazy. He was prone to forgetfulness. His memory got progressively worse over the years. He was unable to keep track of time.

Now that his father was gone, what had once been a punishing and aggravating chore suddenly made him wish he was still alive so he could remind him when to take his meds. What was once a chore had now become an act of filial love and devotion. He broke down crying, upon which a lifetime of pills floated down the stream of his father's life to the final destination of the Sea, the Mother of All Things. Sorrow engulfed him, then he would laugh out loud, relieved that the suffering was now over and he did not have to look after him anymore; then he would be swept up by guilt, only to be overwhelmed again by grief. Finally he cried and cried until the storm subsided. The beeper continued to beep in his hand like a mechanical heart. Beep beep beep... He didn't want to shut it off. He wanted it to beat forever, like his father's heart. Then it stopped all on its own. Never to beep again.

In his final days, my father would sometimes hallucinate or become delusional as he fought for his life. Dad's hallucinations were not always bad. Many of them were quite pleasant, happy and benign. One night, he looked up at the ceiling and said: "Who let in the sky?" It was as if he could see things we could not see. I believe he was actually catching a glimpse of heaven, as if the ceiling of the hospital wall became transparent, revealing a window to God.

WHO LET IN THE SKY?

So the sky did not die with you.
Father, your soul was too light for the heaviness of this world.
I held your balloon string, unwilling to let go.
My grip slipped. I watched your ascent,
weeping as you rose above the storm clouds.
Floating to the sky, you impregnated the Sun.
Golden cascades of light splashed into my eyes, blinding me.
Sunspots burned forever into the retina of my mind's eye.
I could no longer see you.
You are gone. My world is darkness.
But I know you are still here.
I can feel your eternal warmth and kindness.

January 10th, 2010

FIELDS OF HEAVEN

Here I am on the verge again
plowing the cloudy fields of heaven.
I have come to claim my tiny acre of happiness.
Promises of a New World.
A land without borders.
Time and again it has boiled down to this.
What am I to do with so much sky?

Vancouver, 2009

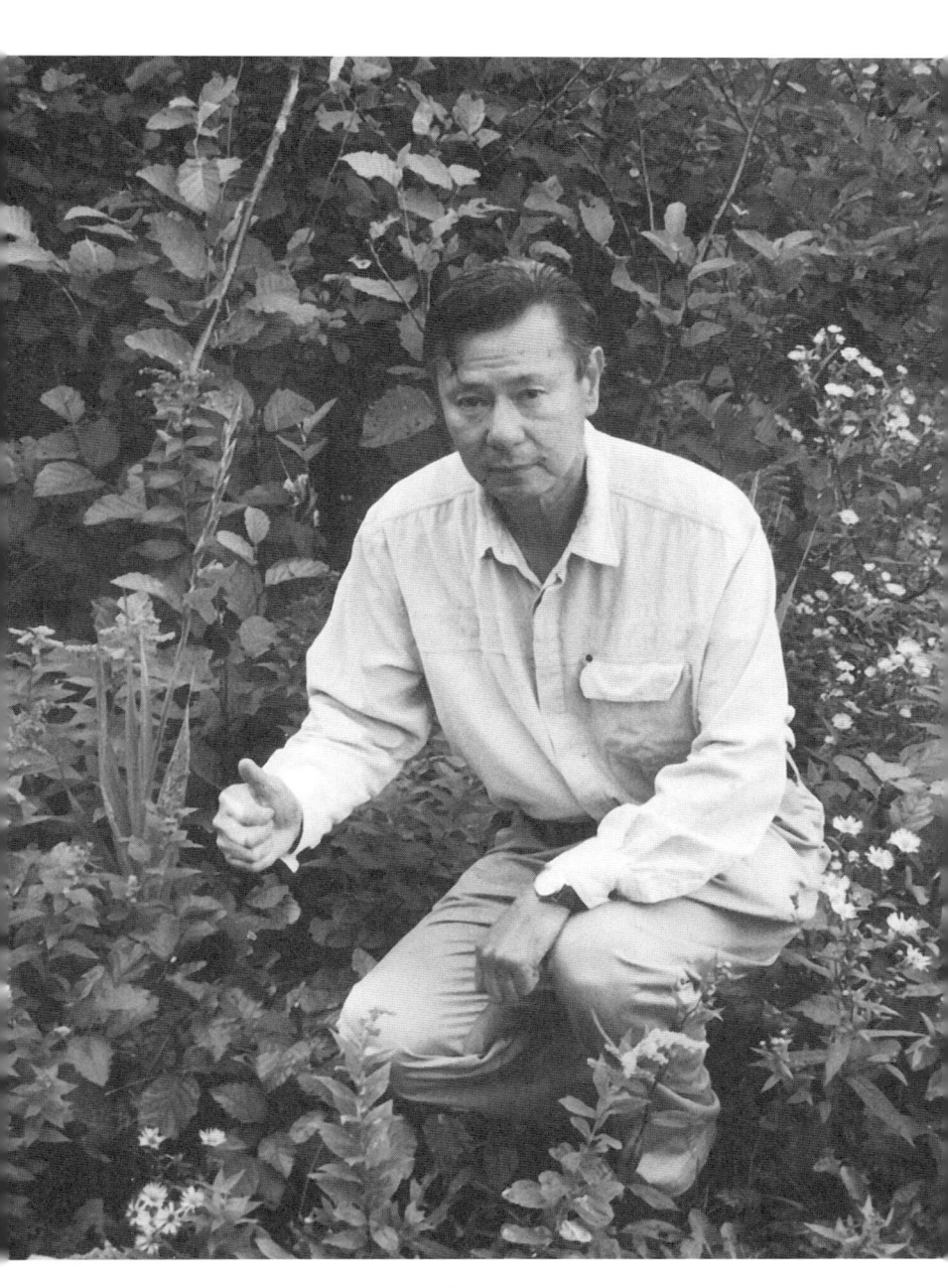

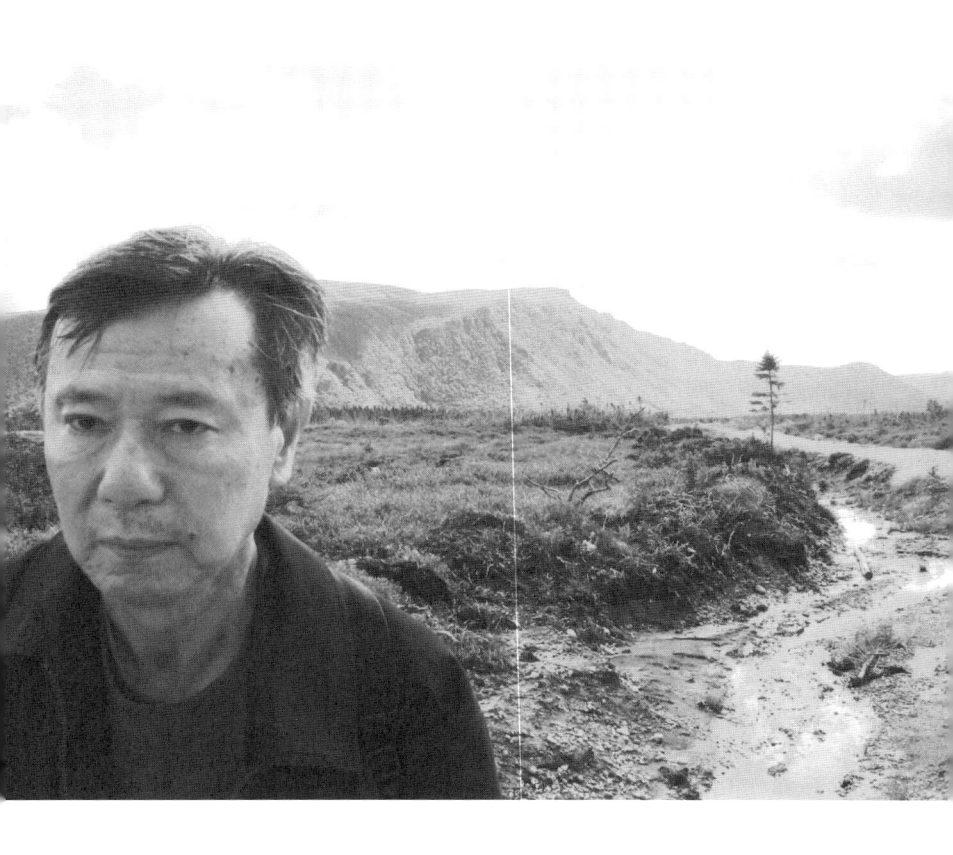

ENTER THE DRAGONFLY

"Out beyond ideas of wrongdoing and rightdoing
there is a field. I'll meet you there.
When the soul lies down in that grass,
the world is too full to talk about.
Ideas, language, even the phrase "each other" doesn't make any sense."

- Rumi

Along the road, I came across a mysterious path that was not on route to where I planned to go. I did not know where it would lead me, but I chose to follow the tug of my heart's bliss. The path opened to a glorious meadow of long grass, glowing golden in the sun. I came across a bench of sturdy varnished wood. Upon it was a plaque that read:

"TO ENJOY THE FLAVOUR
OF LIFE, TAKE BIG BITES."

P.P.F. HAMS

I sat down and leaned back. I took a deep breath, drank in the scenery and basked in the sun's heat. Inspired by the bench's invitation, I retrieved an apple from my packsack and took a hearty crunch into its delicious core. I relished my apple and blessed God for allotting me this tiny acre of happiness. This indeed is heaven on earth to play in the field of the Lord.

Out from yonder, I heard the flutter of mini-propeller wings. To my surprise, a red dragonfly landed on my hand. Its frail rainbow raffia see-through wings quivered in the breeze. The dragonfly's delicate body, perfectly crafted for flight, was evidence of Nature's genius.

"Hello friend. Where did you come from?"

I had a coughing fit, but the dragonfly was not scared off by the commotion and remained faithfully planted on my hand. For some reason this insect trusted me. It knew I would do it no harm. I had made a friend.

Then I noticed the dragonfly's two beady eyes. To my surprise I saw in its eyes a mysterious face staring back at me. I swear it was not my own reflection.

The face looked like my father's.

"Perhaps you are my father reincarnated as a dragonfly, shed the snakeskin of this mortal coil to be reborn as a winged insect?"

That afternoon I confided to my loyal companion as if he was my father, telling him how much I loved him, how much I missed him and hoped that he was happy and free from suffering in his new body.

"You are a magnificent creature! Father, all your life you wanted to be free as a bird. Now your wish has come true. But instead of a bird, you are a dragonfly that can fly free as you want to be."

The dragonfly took my cue and flew away into the golden light of my happy day.

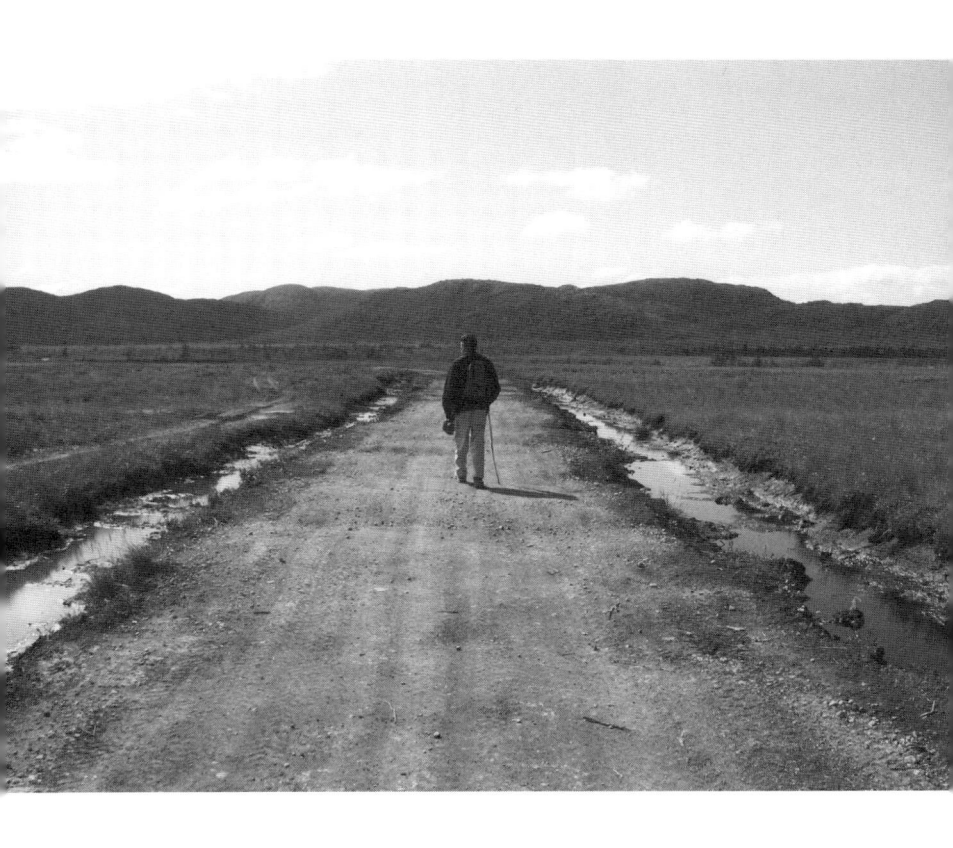

ACKNOWLEDGEMENTS

Special thanks to Jamie Reid, Professor Koh Tai Ann, and my mother Margaret Joyce Wong for editing the manuscript; my brother Kajin Goh for producing the beautiful graphic design of the book. I would like to thank Margaret K. Mitchell, Curtis Steele, and Richard Story for permission to use their photographs; Marni Norwich for her loyal support, appreciation and inspiration in friendship and the writing life. I would like to acknowledge Simon Fraser University's the Writer's Studio participants of 2010, Director Betsy Warland, my amazing Creative Non-Fiction Mentor Ivan Cayote, Eufemia Fantetti, my inspiring fellow Creative Non-Fiction classmates: Cullene Bryant, Esmeralda Cabral, James Gates, Jennifer Irvine, Edward Parker, Kerry Sandomirsky, Peggy Trendell-Jensen and the loving memory of Betty Spinks and Zohreh Ehsani.

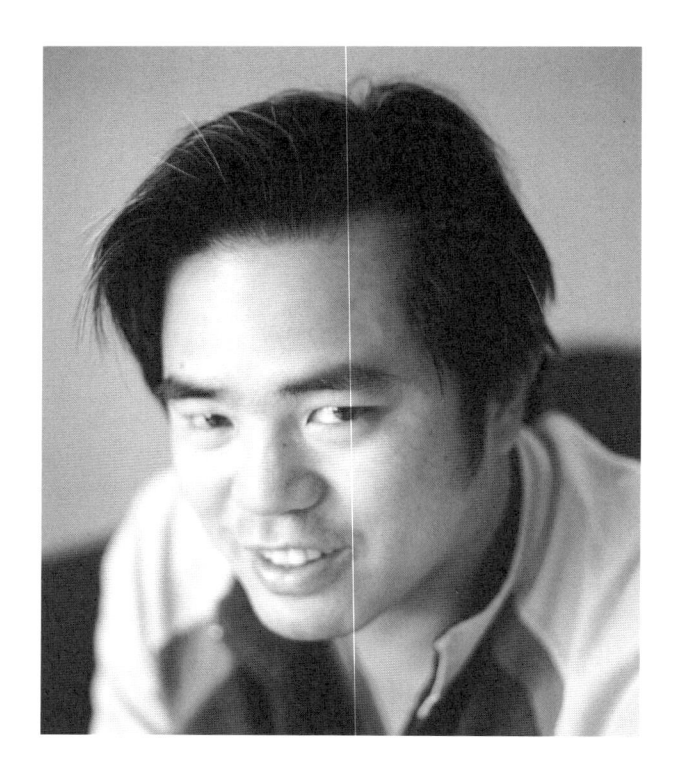

ABOUT THE AUTHOR

Kagan Goh was born in Singapore in 1969. Together with his family, he emigrated to Canada in 1986 and now resides in Vancouver. Kagan was diagnosed with manic depression at 23 in 1993 on Valentine's Day. When his parents took him to see a psychiatrist, he laughed when the symptoms of mania were described to him, thinking they were the positive traits of his personality. Then he was struck with his first depression and he stopped laughing. Over a period of ten years, he suffered several psychotic episodes and a dozen hospitalizations. He started writing about his experiences as therapy and soon became involved in Vancouver's literary community. He became an established spoken word poet who performed at poetry slams, open mics, readings, festivals and radio. His personal mission is to educate people about mental health issues and fight stigma against the mentally ill.

He is an award winning documentary filmmaker, a spoken word poet, novelist, journalist and mental health activist. Kagan's work has been published in *Strike the Wok*, an Asian Canadian anthology of short fiction (TSAR Publications); *Henry Chow and Other Stories from the Asian Canadian Writer's Workshop* (Tradewinds Books) and the Writer's Studio *2010 emerge* (Simon Fraser University). *Who Let In the Sky?* is his first book.

We wish to acknowledge the following authors, publishers, and literary agents for permission to reproduce their work: Alfred Music Publishing Co. Inc for the Lyrics of "Embraceable You" (from "Girl Crazy"), music and lyrics by George Gershwin and Ira Gershwin; David Higham Associates Ltd for "Do Not Go Gentle Into That Good Night" by Dylan Thomas; Coleman Barks for "A Great Wagon", from *The Essential Rumi*, translated by Coleman Barks.